Descending from One Single Line
— Our TCM Culture

《医脉相传—我们的中医药文化》

Chinese-English ‖ 汉英对照

肖莉莉◎著

臧云彩◎中文主审

河南省哲学社会科学规划项目（2018BJY018）、河南省教育厅人文社会科学研究项目（2017-ZZJH-318）、河南中医药大学科研苗圃工程项目（"一带一路"战略视阈下中医药典籍翻译的问题与对策研究）等项目研究成果

全国百佳图书出版单位

时代出版传媒股份有限公司

黄山书社

图书在版编目(CIP)数据

医脉相传：我们的中医药文化 / 肖莉莉著. —合肥：黄山书社，2021.5
ISBN 978-7-5461-5203-5

Ⅰ.①医… Ⅱ.①肖… Ⅲ.①中国医药学-文化 Ⅳ.①R2-05

中国版本图书馆 CIP 数据核字(2021)第 107440 号

医脉相传——我们的中医药文化
YI MAI XIANGCHUAN WOMEN DE ZHONGYIYAO WENHUA

肖莉莉 著

出 品 人	贾兴权
责任编辑	王陶然
责任印制	李 磊
装帧设计	李 昕

出版发行 时代出版传媒股份有限公司(http://www.press-mart.com)
　　　　　黄山书社(http://www.hspress.cn)
地址邮编 安徽省合肥市蜀山区翡翠路1118号出版传媒广场7层 230071
印　　刷 安徽联众印刷有限公司
版　　次 2021年10月第1版
印　　次 2022年2月第2次印刷
开　　本 787mm×1092mm 1/16
字　　数 300千字
印　　张 19.5
书　　号 ISBN 978-7-5461-5203-5
定　　价 55.00元

服务热线　0551-63533706

销售热线　0551-63533761

官方直营书店（https://hsss.tmall.com）

版权所有　侵权必究
凡图书出现印装质量问题，
请与承印厂联系。
联系电话 0551-65661327

序

本书作者肖莉莉从2008年至2011年在北京师范大学外国语言文学学院攻读硕士学位研究生,我是她的学位论文指导教师。肖莉莉从北京师范大学毕业以后,一直从事大学英语教学工作。我与她的联系不多,但知道她一直兢兢业业地从事着教书育人的工作,在教学科研等方面也取得了应有的成绩。

2020年9月,肖莉莉与我联系,说她写了一本汉英对照的中医药方面的书,请我写序。我感到有些惊讶,因为她只是一名大学英语老师,以前并没有中医药方面的学术背景。通过进一步沟通得知,肖莉莉在河南中医药大学入职以后,主动承担了学校在中医药国际传播方面的课程,她希望把自己的英语教学专业与中医药结合起来,并朝这个方向做了不懈的努力。大家现在拿到的这本书就是肖莉莉这些年努力的成果之一。

我本人不懂中医药,不敢对这本书的内容妄加评论,但我知道肖莉莉写这本书很不容易。或者说,谁写这样一本书都不容易。因为懂英语的人很少懂中医药;懂中医药的人未必能用英语写中医药方面的书。本书包括中医的历史、中医基础理论、中医经典著作、历代中医名家、中医诊断学、中药传奇、中国古代医学伦理、中医抗疫史等方面的内容。系统地收集、整理、编撰这些内容已经是一项很大的工程,要完全读懂、深刻把握这些内容绝非易事。尤其是其中不少内容是用文言文表述的,把这些内容准确地翻译为通顺、易懂的英文,更是难上加难了。据我所知,汉英对照的中医学术著作和科普类著作并不是很多。在"讲好中国故事"的背景下,高质量的汉英对照中医学术著作的价值是毋庸置疑的。肖莉莉利用她在英语方面的优势,结合自己积累的中医药方面的知识,写出了这本《医脉相传——我们的中医药文化》,值得表扬。

  有人常说,英语老师只会教英语,没有专业和特长。其实,这是对英语老师的误解。英语老师可以研究语言学、文学、翻译、文化等专业学术领域的问题。英语老师也可以结合自己从事的教学工作以及所在学校的专业特色,开辟新的专业领域。肖莉莉写中医药方面的著作就是一个成功案例。我衷心希望肖莉莉能在这方面走得更远,取得更大的成绩。

  是为序。

程晓堂

2021 年 4 月于北京师范大学

目 录
Contents

第一篇　中医的历史 ··· 1
Section 1　History of TCM
 第一章　萌芽时期 ·· 2
 Chapter 1　Budding Period
 第二章　形成时期 ·· 9
 Chapter 2　Forming Period
 第三章　繁荣时期 ··· 13
 Chapter 3　Booming Period
 第四章　发展时期 ··· 21
 Chapter 4　Developing Period

第二篇　中医基础理论 ··· 26
Section 2　Fundamental Theories of TCM
 第一章　整体观念 ··· 27
 Chapter 1　Holistic View
 第二章　辨证论治 ··· 33
 Chapter 2　Treatment Based on Syndrome Differentiation

第三章　取象比类 …… 37
Chapter 3　Drawing Analogies

第四章　阴阳学说 …… 41
Chapter 4　Theory of Yin-Yang

第五章　五行学说 …… 62
Chapter 5　Theory of the Five Elements

第六章　气血津液 …… 77
Chapter 6　*Qi*, Blood and Body Fluid

第七章　藏象学说 …… 98
Chapter 7　Theory of Visceral Manifestation

第三篇　中医四大经典 …… 105
Section 3　Four Great Classics of TCM

第一章　《黄帝内经》 …… 106
Chapter 1　*Inner Canon of the Yellow Emperor*

第二章　《难经》 …… 111
Chapter 2　*Classic of Medical Difficulties*

第三章　《伤寒杂病论》 …… 113
Chapter 3　*Treatise on Febrile Diseases and Miscellaneous Illnesses*

第四章　《神农本草经》 …… 115
Chapter 4　*Shennong's Classic of Materia Medica*

第四篇　历代中医名家 ·· 118
Section 4　Renowned TCM Doctors in History

第一章　扁鹊 ··· 119
Chapter 1　Bian Que

第二章　华佗 ··· 126
Chapter 2　Hua Tuo

第三章　张仲景 ·· 129
Chapter 3　Zhang Zhongjing

第四章　皇甫谧 ·· 133
Chapter 4　Huangfu Mi

第五章　葛洪 ··· 138
Chapter 5　Ge Hong

第六章　孙思邈 ·· 142
Chapter 6　Sun Simiao

第七章　钱乙 ··· 148
Chapter 7　Qian Yi

第八章　朱震亨 ·· 152
Chapter 8　Zhu Zhenheng

第九章　李时珍 ·· 156
Chapter 9　Li Shizhen

第十章　叶天士 ·· 159
Chapter 10　Ye Tianshi

第五篇　望闻问切 ··· 162
Section 5　Four Diagnostic Methods

第一章　中医诊断学的发展历程 ·· 164
Chapter 1　The Development of TCM Diagnostics

第二章　四诊法 ··· 169
Chapter 2　The Four Diagnostic Methods in TCM

第六篇　中药传奇 ·· 181
Section 6　Legends of Chinese Materia Medica

第一章　白花蛇舌草 ··· 182
Chapter 1　Hedyotis Diffusa

第二章　荜茇 ·· 185
Chapter 2　Piper Longum

第三章　槟榔 ·· 188
Chapter 3　Areca Catechu

第四章　蚕沙 ·· 192
Chapter 4　Silkworm Excrement

第五章　车前草 ··· 198
Chapter 5　Plantain

第六章　穿山龙 ··· 200
Chapter 6　Dioscoreae Nipponicae

第七章 党参 ……………………………………………………………………… 204
Chapter 7　Radix Codonopsis

第八章 地骨皮 …………………………………………………………………… 209
Chapter 8　Cortex Lycii

第九章 地龙 ……………………………………………………………………… 212
Chapter 9　Pheretima

第十章 丁公藤 …………………………………………………………………… 215
Chapter 10　Caulis Erycibes

第十一章 杜鹃花 ………………………………………………………………… 218
Chapter 11　Rhododendron

第十二章 独一味 ………………………………………………………………… 221
Chapter 12　Lamiophlomis Rotata

第十三章 杜仲 …………………………………………………………………… 224
Chapter 13　Eucommia Ulmoides

第十四章 阿胶 …………………………………………………………………… 227
Chapter 14　*Ejiao*

第十五章 茯苓 …………………………………………………………………… 232
Chapter 15　Poria Cocos

第十六章 枸杞子 ………………………………………………………………… 235
Chapter 16　Fructus Lycii

第十七章 桂花 …………………………………………………………………… 238
Chapter 17　Osmanthus Fragrans

第七篇　中国古代医学伦理道德 ………………………………………… 242
Section 7　Medical Ethics in Ancient China

第一章　大医精诚 ……………………………………………………… 243
Chapter 1　On the Absolute Sincerity of Great Doctors

第二章　悬壶济世 ……………………………………………………… 246
Chapter 2　Hanging a Bottle-Gourd to Benefit all Mankind

第三章　杏林春暖 ……………………………………………………… 248
Chapter 3　Apricot Orchard in the Warmth of Spring

第四章　橘井泉香 ……………………………………………………… 251
Chapter 4　Tangerine Leaves and Well Water

第五章　诊宗三昧 ……………………………………………………… 254
Chapter 5　Three Warnings in Practising Medicine

第六章　不为良相,愿为良医 ………………………………………… 256
Chapter 6　Be A Good Prime Minister, or Be A Good Doctor

第八篇　中医千年抗疫史 ………………………………………………… 258
Section 8　TCM Fighting Epidemic with Thousands of Years' History

第一章　先秦时期 ……………………………………………………… 259
Chapter 1　Pre-Qin Period

第二章　两汉三国时期 ………………………………………………… 266
Chapter 2　The Han Dynasties and the Three Kingdoms Period

第三章　魏晋南北朝时期 ··· 270
Chapter 3　Period of the Wei, Jin, and Southern and Northern Dynasties

第四章　唐宋时期 ·· 272
Chapter 4　Period of the Tang and Song Dynasties

第五章　金朝时期 ·· 276
Chapter 5　Period of the Jin Dynasty

第六章　元明清时期 ·· 278
Chapter 6　Period of the Yuan, Ming and Qing Dynasties

第七章　近现代时期 ·· 282
Chapter 7　Period of Modern and Contemporary Times

参考文献 ··· 285
Bibliography

附录1：常见中医典籍名称中英文对照表 ······························· 287
Appendix 1：Common Chinese-English Titles of TCM Classics

附录2：中医常用术语中英文对照表 ······································· 289
Appendix 2：Commonly Used Terminologies of TCM

后记 ··· 299
Afterword

第一篇　中医的历史

习近平主席指出,"中医药学是中国古代科学的瑰宝,也是打开中华文明宝库的钥匙。"中医药博大精深,深深植根于中国传统文化,正如明代杰出医学家张景岳的《类经》序所载:"上极天文,下穷地纪,中悉人事,大而阴阳变化,小而草木昆虫,音律象数之肇端,脏腑经络之曲折。"中医药有数千年的历史,是中国人民长期同疾病做斗争的经验总结。中医药学在古代唯物论和辩证法思想的指导和影响下,通过长期的医疗实践,逐步形成并发展为独特、完整的医学理论体系。

Section 1　History of TCM

As President Xi Jinping pointed out, "Traditional Chinese medicine (also known as TCM) is one of the gems of ancient Chinese science, and it is also the key to open the treasure house of Chinese civilization." Being broad and profound, TCM is deeply rooted in traditional Chinese culture. As Zhang Jingyue, a distinguished physician in the Ming Dynasty (1368 A.D. – 1644 A.D.), wrote in the preface to his book *The Classified Classic* that "TCM provides profound insights into a wide coverage of subjects, ranging from astronomy to geography to human affairs. It not only probes into phenomenon as large as changes of yin-yang, but also thoroughly explores things as small as the growth of trees, blades of grass, vitality of insects, the origin of musical rhymes, the source of emblems and numbers, the subtleties of *zang-fu* organs and the complexity of meridian system in an all-embracing way." TCM, a medical system that has been practiced for thousands of years, has summed up the practice and experience of the Chinese people accumulating in a long course of struggling against diseases. Under the guidance and influence of ancient Chinese materialism and dialectics, TCM has gradually evolved into a medical system with unique and integrated theory through long-term medical practice.

第一章 萌芽时期

中医发展的历史可以分为四个不同的时期。大约在4000年前,中医尚在萌芽阶段,中医就是民间医学。从大约公元前1000年前的中国封建时期到20世纪初,中国的民间医学发展成为系统的中医药体系。

Chapter 1　Budding Period

The history of TCM can be chronologically traced in terms of four different periods. In its infancy about four millennia ago, TCM was, exactly, folk medicine. During China's feudal times lasting from about 1,000 B.C. to the beginning of the 20th century, the folk medicine of China evolved into systematic system of Chinese medicine.

中医的萌芽可以追溯到4000多年前的远古时代。我们的祖先通过寻找食物、狩猎、搭建遮蔽之处保护自己等方式来求得生存。《礼记·礼运》曾记载:"昔者先王未有宫室,冬则居营窟,夏则居橧巢。未有火化,食草木之实、鸟兽之肉,饮其血茹其毛。未有麻丝,衣其羽皮。后圣有作,然后修火之利,范金合土,以为台榭、宫室、牖户。以炮,以燔,以亨,以炙,以为醴酪。治其麻丝,以为布帛。以养生送死,以事鬼神上帝,皆从其朔。"这段话描述了数十万年前的远古时代人类与大自然做斗争的情形,勾勒出原始社会人们从聚木为巢、茹毛饮血,到后来用火烹制食物、以火化腥,用麻丝纺织布帛,并以此养生送死的生活情景。

The history of TCM can be traced back to the primitive period extending back 4,000 years ago. Our ancestors obtained survival through searching plants for food, hunting and building shelters to defend themselves, etc. According to *The Book of Rites*, a historical record compiled some 2,000 years ago, "In remote antiquity, our prehistoric ancestors had no place to live in, hence they sheltered themselves in built caves in winter and wood nests in summer. Since they had no fire to cook the food, they satisfied their hunger with fruits of grass and trees, and with flesh of birds and beasts, drinking their blood, and swallowing their furs and feathers. Due to a lack of linen and silk, they clothed themselves with birds' feathers and animals' hides. The later sovereign arose and got ahead. To seek a better chance of survival, they explored the use of fire, cast metal utensils with models, and burned clay so as to construct terraced buildings, palaces, and make doors and windows. They came up with many ways to make the sweet wine and vinegar inspired by cooking operations of toasting, grilling, boiling and roasting. Flax or silk was interwoven into a linen or silken fabric. All these were going to the source of nourishing the living, making offerings to the dead, and worshipping heaven and earth." This passage depicted the struggle between the ancient people and nature hundreds of thousands of years ago, sketching life scenes of building wood nest, eating the flesh raw and drinking the blood, cooking food over fire, spinning by flax and silk, and nourishing the living and making offerings to the dead.

《韩非子·五蠹》曾记载:"上古之世,人民少而禽兽众,人民不胜禽兽虫蛇;有圣人作,构木为巢,以避群害,而民悦之,使王天下,号之曰有巢氏。民食果蓏蚌蛤,腥臊恶臭而伤腹胃,民多疾病;有圣人作,钻燧取火,以化腥臊,而民说之,使王天下,号之曰燧人氏。"燧人氏钻木取火,火的应用结束了茹毛饮血的时代。

    Records from *Hanfeizi* stated that "In remote antiquity, there were fewer people but more birds and beasts. People could hardly endure the infestations of birds, beasts, insects and snakes any more. A sage then appeared. He gained people's allegiance and was hailed as Youchaoshi to rule the land by building nests in the trees to shun such infestations. During that period, people had no choice but to eat raw foods with fishy and stink smell such as fruits, melons and clams, which impaired the abdomen and stomach, and gave rise to many diseases. Then another sage appeared. He drilled wood to make fire, transforming raw food into cooked food so as to remove the unpleasant smell. Therefore, he became popular with his people and was hailed as Suirenshi to rule the land." Suirenshi's drilling wood to start a fire ended the era of eating the flesh raw and drinking the blood.

毫无疑问,在古人的生活中,火作为热源、光源和燃料发挥了核心作用。用火加热食物,使生食变成熟食,这就是食养、食疗的开端。当古人聚集在火边取暖时,他们很自然地会发现这种热源能立刻有效缓解由于湿寒引起的疼痛,这可能就是能治疗多种疾病的艾灸的起源。火的应用,点燃了灿烂的中医药文明,有着划时代的意义。

There is no doubt that fire played a central role as a source of warmth, light, and fuel in the lives of the ancients. Transforming raw food into cooked food by making a fire to heat the foods made diet therapy possible. As the ancients gathered around fires for warmth, naturally, they would clearly found that the healing powers of heat provided immediate relief for pains caused by cold and dampness-related ailments. This might be the origin of moxibustion, which proved various diseases treating effect. The application of fire ignited the sparks of splendid Chinese medicine civilization, hence it had epoch-making significance.

古人偶然发现一些植物可以治疗某些疼痛,经历了无数次的尝试和失败后,他们逐渐从植物中提取出药物,最终形成了原始中医药学。随着时间的流逝,人们开始主动寻求用砭石疗法、针刺疗法、灸法、汤剂疗法等来预防和治疗疾病。古人在求得基本生存时,难以避免地会受伤。这时,他们很自然地会对受伤的疼痛部位进行按摩。古人发现按压身体的某些穴位会产生各种效果,因此他们开始使用砭石尖锐的一面作为骨针来刺激身体的某些部位以消除疼痛,针灸的初原形式由此诞生。这种疗法逐渐演化为一种针刺疗法,进而形成经络学说。灸法是指人们在点火取暖时用焙热的石块、沙土或草药来进行局部取暖,借以缓解或消除某些病痛。汤剂则是将草药加水浸泡后煎煮内服。汤剂是我国应用最早、最广泛的一种剂型。

The ancient people found, accidentally, that some plants could offer surprising remedies for certain pains. Through countless trials and errors, gradually they came to develop medicines from plants. An embryonic form of primitive herbal medicine was taking shape. With time the ancient people started to take the initiative to prevent and treat diseases by exploring remedies such as stone needle, acupuncture, moxibustion and decoction of herbal medicine. When ancient people strived for basic survival, inevitably there would be injuries. At this time it was natural to react to pain by pressing or rubbing on the injured areas. Ancient people found out that pressing on certain acupoints of the body had a wide variety of effects; hence they began to use sharpened sides of stones as bone needles to stimulate certain parts of the body to eliminate pain. A primitive form of acupuncture was born. Such a treatment gradually evolved into an acupuncture therapeutic system which further developed into the theory of meridians and collaterals. Ancient people created moxibustion therapy to relieve or alleviate pain by heated stones, sand or baking herbs for local heating when they lit a fire for warmth. To drink one decoction of herbal medicine, one normally had to soak all the herbs in water before decocting the mixture of herbs and water for internal use. As a common remedy, a decoction of herbal medicine is the earliest and widely used medicament in China.

神农氏,即炎帝,是历史传说中上古的帝王。上古传说中有"三皇五帝"之说,这其中"三皇"指的就是伏羲氏、神农氏和燧人氏。事实上,神农氏只是一个部落的首领,由于有独特的贡献,才被尊称为炎帝。

Shennongshi, also known as Emperor Yan (the Fiery Emperor), was a legendary Chinese ruler in pre-dynastic times. The origin of Emperor Yan (the Fiery Emperor) was a legend of ancient sovereigns known as the Three Sovereigns and Five Emperors. It was said that the Three Sovereigns were Fuxi, Shennong and Suiren. Actually, Shennongshi was merely a tribal leader, and he was honored as Emperor Yan (the Fiery Emperor) due to his unique contributions.

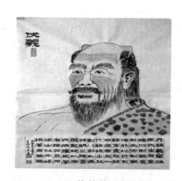 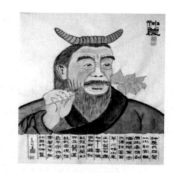

伏羲像　　　　　　　　　神农像
Portrait of Fuxi　　　　　Portrait of Shennong

关于中草药的发现和运用,一般都认为起源于神农氏。在古代,有"神农尝百草,一日遇七十毒"的故事。相传神农人身牛首,但极具爱心。他发现许多百姓被病痛折磨着,就走遍天下,采集草药,并依据草药的不同性质给病人服用相应的草药。为了进一步了解药性,神农亲自品尝了上百种草药。据说神农仅仅在一天当中,就遇到了 70 种有毒的植物,所以又被称为"药王神"。

It is widely acknowledged that the discovery and application of herbal medicine originated from Shennongshi. In ancient times, there was a story of "Shennong tasting a hundred herbs and meeting 70 poisons a day". Shennong was said to have been born with the head of a bull and the body of a man, but he was a loving man. Shennong found that many people had been tortured by illnesses, so he traveled all over the country, collecting herbs and giving away to the sick according to their different properties. Shennong tasted a hundred herbs daily to assess their qualities. He was said to have been poisoned 70 times in one single day during his investigations. Hence he was also known as "the God of Medicine".

在中国神话中,神农尝遍百草,以身试药,发明了用草药治疗疾病的方法,这便是中医药的起源。清代陈元龙编撰的《格致镜原》曾载:"神农尝百草,一日而遇七十毒,得茶以解之。"

In Chinese mythology, Shennong tasted a hundred herbs, tried the medicine by himself, and invented a way for treating diseases with herbs. This was how Chinese medicine started. Chen Yuanlong, a celebrity in the Qing Dynasty (1644 A.D.–1911 A.D.), said in his *Gezhi Jingyuan* that "Shennong tasted a hundred herbs and came across 70 poisons a day, but was detoxified with tea."

中国的饮茶文化可以追溯到神农所处的新石器时代,当时茶叶被用作草药。中国人发现茶,由"神农尝百草,一日而遇七十毒,得茶以解之"而起。神农尝百草多次中毒,都多亏了茶解毒。

The drinking of tea in China could be traced back to the times of Shennong during the Neolithic Age, and at that time tea leaves were used as medicinal herbs. The Chinese people attribute the origins of tea to the legend that "Shennong tasted a hundred of herbs, met 70 poisons in a single day, and he came upon tea as an antidote." Shennong was poisoned for many times, all thanks to the tea detoxification.

有一天,神农在采药时,尝到一种草叶,顿时头晕目眩、口干舌麻。这时,一阵风吹过,他闻到一种清新的香味,但他不知道那香味来自哪里。他发现树上有几片叶子缓缓落下,便心生好奇,拾起一片放入口中咀嚼。那叶子的味道虽然苦涩,但有清香回甘之味,让他口齿生津,精神振奋,头晕目眩之感减轻,口干舌麻之症渐消。神农便将这种叶子定名为"茶",这就是茶的最早发现,也是有关中国饮茶起源最普遍的说法。

One day, Shennong tasted a leaf when collecting herbs. Suddenly he felt dizzy with suspected poisoning symptoms such as dry mouth and numb tongue. At this time, he smelt a kind of fresh fragrance when a gust of wind blew, but he did not know where was the fragrance from. He found several leaves falling down from a tree slowly. Being curious, he picked up one leaf and put it in his mouth to chew. Although it was bitter, it had enduring fragrance and unforgettable aftertaste which engendered the secretion of saliva and made him in high spirits. He felt less dizzy and the dryness and numbness gradually vanished. Hence Shennong gave this kind of leave the name "*cha*" (*tea*). This was the earliest discovery of tea and the most common saying about the origin of tea drinking in China.

药膳的产生归功于神农。中国的药膳源远流长,据《淮南子·修务训》记载:"(神农)尝百草之滋味,水泉之甘苦,令民知所辟就。当此之时,一日而遇七十毒。"这反映了早在远古时代,中华民族就开始探索食物和药物的功用。"知所辟就",就是让百姓知道百草、水泉的性能和滋味,避其毒性,合理取用。这就是中医特色概念"药食同源"的最早缘起,为后世本草学的形成和药膳食疗的发展奠定了基础。"神农尝百草,始有医药""药食同源"的传说反映了那个时期的特征。

Chinese medicated diet, which dated back to ancient times, owed its existence to Shennong. According to *The Necessity of Training: Huainanzi*, "Shennong tasted a hundred herbs daily to assess their qualities, and identified the sweetness and bitterness of water sources. He taught people to shun risks in usage of herbs. Once he accidentally poisoned himself 70 times in a single day." This ancient legend of Shennong reflected that early in remote antiquity the Chinese nation began to explore functions of food and medicine. "To shun risks" here is to avoid toxicity and to seize the rational use of properties of herbs together with the tastes of springs. This is the earliest origin of the TCM characterized concept—"medicine and food sharing the same source", which lays the groundwork for the formation of materia medica and the development of the medicated diet therapy. Sayings like "Shennong tasting a hundred herbs" and "medicine and food steming from the same source" reflect the characteristic of that period.

第二章 形成时期

中医绵延数千年,在其漫长的进程中,夏朝时期酒精的发现和商朝时期中药汤剂的出现都堪称中医史上的飞跃。在已出土的殷商时期甲骨文中,发现了大量关于疾病的名称。在那个时期,医巫并存,卜筮史料中记载了大量的医药卫生方面的内容,形成了医学的雏形。随着生产力的发展,社会分工日趋专业化,医巫逐渐分离,专职医生出现。据《周礼·天官》记载,西周时期对医学进行了分科,分为食医(膳食营养医生)、疾医(内科医生)、疡医(外科医生)和兽医,这是我国乃至世界上最早的医学分科。

Chapter 2　Forming Period

TCM has stretched for thousands of years of history. During its long course, the discovery of alcohol in the Xia Dynasty (2070 B.C.-1600 B.C.) and the first appearance of herbal decoction in the Shang Dynasty (1600 B.C.-1046 B.C.) were both big leaps. On the unearthed oracle bone inscriptions of the Shang Dynasty, lots of disease names were discovered. Doctors and witch doctors coexisted at that time, and large amounts of information about medicine and health was found in the historical materials of divination, which indicated that early medicine began to take shape. With the development of productive forces, the social division of labor mounted to an increasing high level of specialization. Doctors and witch doctors were gradually separated and a group of specialist appeared. The earliest medical division of China was recorded in *Rites of Zhou*: *Officer of Heaven* in which doctors fell into four categories during the Western Zhou Dynasty (1046 B.C.-771 B.C.): dietician, physician, surgeon and veterinarian. These were the earliest medical branches in China and even in the world.

《周礼·天官·冢宰》详细记载了当时的分工情形:"医师掌医之政令,聚毒药以共医事。凡邦之有疾病者,有疕疡者造焉,则使医分而治之。岁终,则稽其医事,以制其食","食医掌和王之六食、六饮、六膳、百羞、百酱、八珍之齐。凡食齐视春时,羹齐视夏时,酱齐视秋时,饮齐视冬时","疾医掌养万民之疾病。四时皆有疠疾:春时有痟首疾,夏时有痒疥疾,秋时有疟寒疾,冬时有嗽上气疾。以五味、五谷、五药养其病,以五气、五声、五色视其死生,两之以九窍之变,参之以九藏之动","疡医掌肿疡、溃疡、金疡、折疡之祝药,劀、杀之齐。凡疗疡,以五毒攻之,以五气养之,以五药疗之,以五味节之","兽医掌疗兽病,疗兽疡。凡疗兽病,灌而行之,以节之,以动其气,观其所发而养之。凡疗兽疡,灌而劀之,以发其恶,然后药之、养之、食之。凡兽之有病者、有疡者,使疗之。死则计其数以进退之。"从以上的记载得知,早在2000多年前,我国的医学分科已经分工明确,十分缜密。

Rites of Zhou: *Officer of Heaven* gave a detailed record of such division at that time, "Doctors took charge of medical decree and TCM drugs collection for medical use. Anyone who suffered from internal diseases or traumatism could come to receive treatment. Treatment options and assignment of duties depended on the severity of the patients conditions. A year-end assessment of doctors would decide their salary distribution", "Dietician was responsible for the emperor's daily intake of staples, drinks, meats, delicious foods, foods tailored to sauce products and other precious delicacies. Cereals should be prepared as warm as spring, soup as hot as summer, sauces as cool as autumn and drinks as cold as winter", "Physician held responsible for diseases of the masses. Epidemic diseases occurred all year round: headaches in spring, scabies in summer, malaria and aversion to cold in autumn, and cough and asthma in winter. Doctors performed treatment by adoption of five flavors, five grains and five herbs. The five odors, five voices and five colors were criteria for whether the treatment would be carried on. The open and close of the patients' nine orifices (two eyes, two nostrils, two ears, mouth, external genitalia and anal opening) and the conditions of the nine viscera (liver, heart, spleen, lung, kidney, stomach, large intestine, small intestine and bladder) would be examined for diagnosis", "Surgeons bore the responsibility for abscesses, ulcers, metal wounds and traumata by medicine for external application and removal of pus and slough. Abscess treatment demanded five kinds of strong medicine to dissipate it, the five cereals to nurse it, five sorts of mild medicine to cure it and five flavors to adjust it", "Veterinarians had charge of treatment of livestock. They washed their body and performed livestock-walking to invigorate the circulation of blood for the purpose of controlling the diseases. Symptoms were examined carefully for a better cure and ways of cleaning the wounds, removing the slough to dissipate the poison for the livestock's abscesses were developed. The veterinarians then applied medicine to them, nursed them and fed them. All the livestock with internal and traumatic diseases could receive medical treatment. Salaries and positions of the veterinarians rest with the figures in its cumulative number of death cases of the livestock." From the above records, medical division of China two thousand years ago was marked by a clear division and meticulous arrangements.

春秋时期，秦国医和提出了"六气病源"学说。据《左传·昭公元年》记载："天有六气，降生五味，发为五色，徵为五声。淫生六疾。六气曰阴、阳、风、雨、晦、明也。分为四时，序为五节，过则为菑，阴淫寒疾，阳淫热疾，风淫末疾，雨淫腹疾，晦淫惑疾，明淫心疾。"这是关于"六气病源"学说最早的记载。事实上，《黄帝内经》才系统阐述了"风、寒、暑、湿、燥、火"六气学说。

During the Spring and Autumn Period, a doctor named Yi He from the State of Qin raised the "source of the disease resulting from six *qi*" theory. Records of the six *qi* in the natural world (yin, yang, wind, rain, night and day) could be found in *Chronicle of Zuo*, "The six *qi* descend to develop five flavors, manifesting as five colors, and fulfilling as five sounds of *gong*, *shang*, *jiao*, *zheng* and *yu* by which the ancient Chinese people used to mark the musical sound. Anything excessive may lead to six diseases. Six *qi* (yin, yang, wind, rain, night and day) manifest as the four seasons and array as the rhythm of five sounds. Anything in excess may give rise to health problems. Excessive yin may lead to cold disease, excessive yang to hot disease, excessive wind to limbs disease, and excessive dampness of rain to stomach disease. Staying up too late may cause delusions, and worrying beyond measure may cause heart diseases. " This was the earliest record of the "source of the disease resulting from six *qi*". Actually, it was not until the coming out of *Inner Canon of the Yellow Emperor* that the theory of six-*qi* (wind, cold, summer-heat, dampness, dryness and heat) was systematically elaborated.

春秋战国时期,一位名叫扁鹊的传奇般的医学家提出了中医四诊法,即望、闻、问、切,奠定了中医诊断治疗的基础。

During the Spring and Autumn Period (770 B.C.-476 B.C.) and the Warring States Period (475 B.C.-221 B.C.), Bian Que, a legendary Chinese medical scientist, put forward the four diagnostic methods—inspection, auscultation and olfaction, inquiry, pulse-taking and palpation, thus laying the groundwork for TCM diagnosis and treatment.

中医四大经典,即《黄帝内经》《难经》《伤寒杂病论》和《神农本草经》。这些医学典籍的问世,标志着中医学理论体系的初步形成。

The coming out of *Inner Canon of the Yellow Emperor*, *Classic of Medical Difficulties*, *Treatise on Febrile Diseases and Miscellaneous Illnesses* and *Shennong's Classic of Materia Medica*, which are known in TCM as the four great classics, marks the initial shape of theoretical system of TCM.

秦汉时期,中国现存最早的中医理论巨著《黄帝内经》构建了中医药学的理论框架,是中医发展史上的里程碑,标志着临床实践的积累向系统理论总结的转变,初步奠定了中医药学的理论基础。

During the Qin and Han Dynasties (221 B.C.-220 A.D.), the earliest extant TCM monumental masterpiece *Inner Canon of the Yellow Emperor* established the theoretical framework of Chinese medicine, thus standing out as a notable landmark in the progress of TCM and marking the transformation from the accumulation of clinical practice to the systematic summary of TCM doctors' know-what and know-how, which provided a theoretical basis for TCM.

第三章　繁荣时期

汉朝以后,中医学进入繁荣时期。东汉时期张仲景编著的《伤寒杂病论》提出了治疗温病的原则和方法,确立了中医辨证论治的诊疗原则和方法,是我国第一部临床医学专著,为我国临床医学的发展铺平了道路。

Chapter 3　Booming Period

After the Han Dynasty (202 B.C.-220 A.D.), TCM was entering a new period of full bloom with the result that *Treatise on Febrile Diseases and Miscellaneous Illnesses*, compiled by Zhang Zhongjing in the Eastern Han Dynasty (25 A.D.-220 A.D.), put forward the principles and methods of diagnosis and treatment for warm diseases. This classic, which is the first clinical medicine monograph in China, establishes the principles and methodology for diagnosis and treatment based on syndrome differentiation, thus paving the way for the development of clinical medicine in our country.

同时期出现了另一部医学经典巨著《神农本草经》,提出了单行、相须、相使、相畏、相恶、相反、相杀等"七情和合"的药物配伍理论,为组方提供了重要的理论依据,是我国现存最早的药物学专著,为中药学理论的形成和发展奠定了基础。

Another monumental work of this period was *Shennong's Classic of Materia Medica*, in which it incorporated the theory of the compatibility of medicinal ingredients—"seven relations", acting singly, mutual reinforcement, mutual assistance, mutual counteraction, mutual inhibition, mutual opposition and mutual suppression, thus providing theoretical basis for formula-forming theory with drugs, and establishing the foundation for the formation and development of Chinese materia medica theory as the earliest extant classic on materia medica in China.

东汉末期,中医学发展很快,名医涌现,华佗就是其中之一。华佗精通内、外、妇、儿、针灸各科,尤其擅长外科手术。据记载,华佗是世界上第一个在外科手术中使用麻醉药的人。

The rapid progress in TCM in the late years of the Eastern Han Dynasty brought up lots of renowned doctors. Hua Tuo was one of them. Hua Tuo was proficient in internal medicine, surgery, gynecology, pediatrics and acupuncture, especially good at surgery. He was recorded to be the first person to use anesthetic during surgery in the world.

三国时期,竹林七贤之一、魏国名士嵇康的《养生论》是中国古代第一篇较全面、系统的养生专论,对后世养生思想产生了深远的影响。

During the Three Kingdoms Period (220 A.D.-280 A.D.), *Essay on Health Cultivation* by Ji Kang, one of the Seven Sages of the Bamboo Grove, a celebrity of the State of Wei, was the first comparatively comprehensive and systematic masterpiece on health cultivation in ancient China, exerting a far-reaching impact on the thoughts of health cultivation for future generations.

西晋太医令王叔和所著《脉经》系统阐述了24种脉象,成为我国现存最早的脉学专著。西晋时期,皇甫谧撰成《针灸甲乙经》一书,为我国现存最早的一部针灸学专著。书中详尽论述有关脏腑、经络等理论,对后世针灸医学的发展有很大的影响,经络理论和针灸学说就此形成。东晋时期,葛洪著有《肘后备急方》一书,向民众普及针灸知识。

The Pulse Classic, compiled by an imperial medical official Wang Shuhe during the Western Jin Dynasty (265

A.D. -316 A.D.), was the earliest extant monograph specializing in sphygmology in China in which 24 pulse conditions were systematically expounded. Compiled by Huangfu Mi during the Western Jin Dynasty, *A-B Canon of Acupuncture and Moxibustion*, which expounded on the theories of *zang-fu* organs and meridians and collaterals, was the earliest extant work on acupuncture and moxibustion in China and had a huge impact on the development of acupuncture and moxibustion for future generations. Thus the theories of meridians and collaterals, and acupuncture and moxibustion had been in place. During the Eastern Jin Dynasty (317 A.D. -420 A.D.), Ge Hong compiled *Handbook of Prescriptions for Emergencies*, popularizing knowledge of acupuncture and moxibustion to the masses.

隋朝巢元方主持编撰的《诸病源候论》对内、外、妇、儿科等疾病作了详尽的描述,载列证候1739条,是我国最早的病因证候学专著。

Treatise on Causes and Symptoms of Diseases, compiled under the leadership of Chao Yuanfang in the Sui Dynasty (581 A.D. -618 A.D.), was the first extant monumental monograph on pathogenic symptomatology in China. It gave a detailed description of 1,739 syndromes ranging from internal medicine, surgery, gynecology to pediatrics, etc.

《唐本草》,亦称《唐·新修本草》,有时简称《新修本草》,是唐高宗显庆四年(公元659年)苏静等人以唐朝政府名义集体编修的药典,这是中国第一部由政府颁布的药典,也是世界上最早的药典。

Materia Medica of Tang Dynasty, also known as *The Newly-Revised Materia Medica of Tang Dynasty*, *The Newly-Revised Materia Medica* for short, collectively compiled by Su Jing and other medical practitioners under the name of the government in the year of 659 A.D., was not only the first national pharmacopoeia issued by the government in China, but the earliest pharmacopoeia in the world.

唐朝重视医学教育。公元 624 年,中央在长安设立太医署。太医署具有行政、教学和医疗职能,由行政、教学、医疗、药工四大部分组成,太医署是我国第一所由国家开办的颇具影响的医学校。

Medical education rose to importance during the Tang Dynasty（618 A.D.-907 A.D.）. In the year of 624 A.D., the Bureau of Imperial Physicians was established in the capital city of Chang'an（now Xi'an）with the functional roles in administration, teaching and medical practice. The bureau, which consisted of four sections—administration, teaching, medical practice and pharmaceuticals, was the earliest influential medical institution organized by the government in ancient China.

孙思邈是唐朝著名的医药学家,他编纂了《备急千金要方》和《千金翼方》两部医学经典,共记载 6000 多个药方,总结了中国自古以来至唐初的医学成就。这两部典籍堪称中医学发展史上的里程碑。孙思邈因其杰出的成就被后人尊称为"药王"。孙思邈还提出习医之人要兼有医术精湛、医德高尚两个方面。他在《大医精诚》一文中提出两者兼备才是道德观的体现。这一核心价值观得到了中医药界的自觉维护。

Sun Simiao, a celebrated medical expert in the Tang Dynasty, compiled two TCM classics, *Prescriptions Worth a Thousand Pieces of Gold for Emergencies* and *Supplement to Prescriptions Worth a Thousand Pieces of Gold*, which recorded more than 6,000 prescriptions and was a sum-up of medical achievements from ancient times to the early Tang Dynasty. Both are recognized as representative Chinese medicine milestone works in the development of Chinese medicine. Sun Simiao is honored by later generations as "the King of Herbal Medicine". He proposes that both proficient medical skills and lofty medical ethics are indispensable for TCM practitioners. In his *On the Absolute Sincerity of Great Doctors*, Sun Simiao puts forward that a twin emphasis of both contributes to the embodiment of moral values. Such core value is upheld by the TCM circles conscientiously.

宋朝时期,政府尤为重视医学教育,设立了太医局、药局、方剂局等医疗机构。作为培养中医人才的最高机构,太医局培训教育医学人员。公元 1057 年,又成立了校正医书局,校正、核对、编撰医学知识。

During the Song Dynasty (960 A.D.-1279 A.D.), medical education became a more focused issue for the government. Medical institutions such as China's Imperial Medical Bureau, Bureau for Medicine and Bureau for Prescription sprung up in succession. As the highest TCM talent training organization, China's Imperial Medical Bureau was authorized to perform its duties in training and educating qualified medical practitioners. In 1057 A.D., Bureau for Revising Medical Books was set up, proofreading, checking and compiling medical knowledge.

金元时期,涌现出许多医学流派,其中最具代表性的是"金元四大家":刘完素、张从正、李杲和朱震亨。这四大流派极大地丰富和发展了中医学理论。刘完素以"火热"立论,认为"火热"为主要病因,强调外感"六气皆从火化"及"五志过极皆能生火",临床用药以寒凉为主,被后世称为"寒凉派",其学术思想对后世影响很大。张从正主张"六气"致病,病由邪生,"邪去则正安",故治病当以祛邪为要旨。他提倡临床使用"汗、吐、下"三法攻邪治病,后世称之为"攻下派"。李杲则提出了"内伤脾胃,百病由生"的观点,认为脾胃乃元气之本,疾病的发生多与脾胃损伤有关,临床多以补益脾胃为主,后世称之为"补土派"。朱震亨倡导"相火论",认为"阳常有余,阴常不足",临床主张滋阴降火,被后世称为"滋阴派"。这些流派建树颇多,对后世医学的发展影响很大。

During the Jin Dynasty (1115 A.D.-1234 A.D.) and the Yuan Dynasty (1271 A.D.-1368 A.D.), numerous medical schools sprung up all over the country. Out of these schools, the most representative were the "Four Great Medical Scientists of the Jin and Yuan Dynasties", namely, Liu Wansu, Zhang Congzheng, Li Gao and Zhu Zhenheng. These four medical schools greatly enriched and developed TCM theories. Basing his argument squarely on his study of "fire-heat", Liu Wansu believed that "fire-heat" was the main cause of diseases. He stressed that "exogenously contracted six climatic factors may all transform into fire" and "extreme hyperactivity of the five emotions can all give rise to fire". Drugs cold and cool were a top priority for clinical treatment. Hence his theory was known as the school of "cold and cool", which had huge impact on later generations. Zhang Congzheng deemed that the occurrence of disease was mainly caused by invasion of exogenous pathogenic qi. "As long as such pathogenic qi was driven out, the disease would naturally disappear." Therefore clinical treatment was aimed at eliminating the pathogenic qi, which should be removed through "diaphoresis, emesis and purgation". Hence his theory was known as the school of "purgation". Li Gao expressed his opinion that "internal impairment of spleen and stomach gives rise to various diseases". Spleen and stomach were the basis of original qi, therefore the occurrence of disease was mostly related to the impairment of the spleen and stomach. In clinical treatment, he underlined the importance of tonifying and invigorating the spleen and stomach, hence he was regarded as the founder of the school of "reinforcing the earth". Zhu Zhenheng was a strong advocate of the "ministerial fire" theory. He believed that "yang is usually excessive while yin is always deficient" and inclined to adopt the remedies of nourishing yin and reducing fire in clinical practice. Hence he was regarded by later generations as the school of "nourishing yin". These schools yielded fruitful results which exerted a tremendous influence on the medical development of later ages.

明清时期是中医理论的系统整理和发展阶段。这一时期，许多医学专家对前人的医学著作和经验进行了整理和分类，进一步发展和深化了中医理论。

The Ming and Qing Dynasties (1368 A.D. – 1911 A.D.) were characterized by systematic sorting out and developing of TCM theories. During this period, many medical specialists sorted and classified the medical works and experiences of their predecessors, which took TCM theories a step further.

明朝最著名的医学家李时珍最大的成就是撰成不朽的巨著《本草纲目》，全书共有 52 卷，是推动中医药理论发展的药学史上的里程碑。《本草纲目》被翻译成多国语言，英国博物学家、生物学家达尔文称这本书为"中国古代百科全书",该书所取得的成就使其在全世界范围内广受欢迎。

The most famous medical expert of the Ming Dynasty was Li Shizhen, whose most incredible achievement was his monumental masterpiece—*Compendium of Materia Medica*, which consisted of 52 volumes at the time of its printing. It served as a landmark in TCM pharmaceutical history in the progress of TCM theories. This book has been translated into many languages. Charles Robert Darwin, the British naturalist and biologist, author of 1859's *On the Origin of Species*, hailed the book as an "ancient Chinese encyclopedia". The remarkable achievement has won it popularity throughout the world.

明朝时期,由明朝的开国皇帝朱元璋的第五个儿子朱橚主持编撰的《普济方》是我国现存的最大的一部方书。

During the Ming Dynasty, *Formulary of Universal Relief*, compiled under the leadership of Zhu Su, the fifth son of Zhu Yuanzhang(the first emperor of the Ming Dynasty), was the extant largest medical formulary in China.

明末汪昂所撰《汤头歌诀》收载方歌200余首,至今仍是医学启蒙的必读书目之一。

During the late Ming Dynasty, *Rhyming Versified Prescriptions* by Wang Ang collected approximately 200 rhyming versified prescriptions, serving as a must-read for medical enlightenment so far.

明清时期,温病学说的形成与发展是中医学理论的一大突破。明代医学家吴又可所著《温疫论》一书,认为温疫的病原"非风非寒非暑非湿,乃天地间别有一种异气所感",提出了"戾气"学说。《温疫论》是中国历史上第一部系统研究急性传染病的医学著作。至清代,中医在温病的治疗方面积累了丰富经验。著名温病学家叶天士著有《温热论》,创立了温热病的卫气营血辨证理论,制定了预防和治疗温病的原则和方法,代表了中医药防治温病的理论和实践成果。温病学的其他代表作还有薛雪的《湿热条辨》、吴瑭的《温病条辨》

和王士雄的《温热经纬》等，温病学是我国人民长期与外感热病做斗争的经验总结。

During the Ming and Qing Dynasties, the formation and development of the theory of warm diseases marked a quantum leap in TCM theories. In the *Treatise on Pestilence* by Wu Youke, a distinguished physician in the Ming Dynasty, he produced the theory of "pestilential qi", holding that the cause of pestilence was "pestilent qi rather than wind, cold, summer-heat and dampness between heaven and earth". *Treatise on Pestilence* was the first medical book centering around systematic study of acute infectious disease in China. By the Qing Dynasty, TCM practitioners had accumulated rich experiences in treating warm diseases. *Treatise on Warm Febrile Diseases* by Ye Tianshi during the Qing Dynasty created the therapies for warm febrile diseases based on syndrome differentiation system by adopting the defensive, qi, nutritive and blood as a theoretical model. Also he formulated the principles and methods for prevention and treatment of warm diseases which were regarded as a representative of the theory and achievements of TCM practice in this field. Other representative works were *Treatise on Differentiation and Treatment of Dampness-Heat Diseases* by Xue Xue, *Treatise on Differentiation and Treatment of Warm Diseases* by Wu Tang, and *An Outline of Warm-Heat Diseases* by Wang Shixiong, etc. The theory of warm disease served as a summation of experiences of the Chinese people in the long-term struggle against exogenous pathogenic heat diseases.

第四章　发展时期

中国政府一贯重视中医药的发展。中华人民共和国成立后,中医药的发展进入了一个新阶段。政府制定了一系列保护、扶持、促进中医药发展的方针政策。

Chapter 4　Developing Period

Chinese government has all along attached importance to the development of TCM. After the founding of the People's Republic of China, TCM has advanced to a new stage. The government has formulated a series of policies and guidelines to protect, support and promote the development of TCM.

中华人民共和国成立初期,把"团结中西医"作为我国三大卫生工作方针之一,确立了中医药的地位和作用。

During the early days of the People's Republic of China, the government put a high value on integrating traditional Chinese and Western medicine as one of its three guidelines for health work, establishing the status and role of TCM.

1969年,中国政府启动"523"项目,研究抗疟防治药物,屠呦呦担任中药抗疟组组长。

In 1969, the Chinese government launched National Malaria Project "523", an antimalarial medicine research mission, and Tu Youyou served as the leader of the anti-malaria team of TCM.

1978年,中共中央转发卫生部党组《关于认真贯彻党的中医政策,解决中医队伍后继乏人问题的报告》,大力支持中医药事业的发展。1986年,国务院成立相对独立的中医药管理部门。

In 1978, the Communist Party of China (CPC) Central Committee transmitted the document of "Report on Implementing the Party's Policies Regarding TCM and Cultivating TCM Practitioners" issued by the Party Group of Ministry of Health, strongly supporting the development of TCM. In 1986, the State Council established a relatively independent administration of TCM.

为了进一步推进和确保中医药的发展,国务院于2003年和2009年分别颁发了《中华人民共和国中医药条例》和《国务院关于扶持和促进中医药事业发展的若干意见》,逐步形成了较为完善的中医药政策体系。

In order to further carry forward and ensure the development of TCM, in 2003 and 2009, the State Council issued the "Regulations of the People's Republic of China on Traditional Chinese Medicine" and the "Opinions on Supporting and Promoting the Development of Traditional Chinese Medicine" respectively. A relatively complete policy system of TCM gradually takes shape.

2015年,国务院常务会议通过《中医药法(草案)》,为中医药的发展提供法制保障。2016年,国务院印发《中医药发展战略规划纲要(2016-2030年)》,把中医药发展上升为国家战略。同年,国务院新闻办公室发表《中国的中医药》白皮书,这是中国政府首次就中医药发展发表白皮书。2016年底,中共中央、国务院印发《"健康中国2030"规划纲要》,提出了一系列振兴中医药发展的任务和举措。中医药事业进入新的历史发展时期。

In 2015, the executive meeting of the State Council passed "the Law on Traditional Chinese Medicine (Draft)", providing legal guarantee for TCM development. In 2016, with the rise of TCM development for national strategy, the State Council issued "the Outline of the Strategic Plan on the Development of Traditional Chinese

Medicine (2016–2030)". Later that year, China's State Council Information Office issued a white paper titled "Traditional Chinese Medicine in China", which was the first white paper on the development of TCM in China released by the Chinese government. The CPC Central Committee and the State Council released "the Outline of the Healthy China 2030 Plan" by the end of 2016, putting forward a string of tasks and measures to revitalize TCM development. TCM development entered into a new historical period.

2015年,中国科学家屠呦呦因发现青蒿素治疗疟疾的新疗法获诺贝尔生理学或医学奖。她是第一位在该领域获得诺贝尔科学奖项的华人女性科学家。青蒿素的发现挽救了全球数百万人的生命,尤其是在发展中国家。

In 2015, Chinese scientist Tu Youyou won the Nobel Prize for the discovery of artemisinin, an anti-malaria drug. She is the first Chinese woman to win the Nobel Prize in Physiology or Medicine. The discovery of artemisinin has saved millions of people's lives on the planet, especially in developing countries.

屠呦呦在瑞典卡罗林斯卡医学院发表题为《青蒿素——中医药给世界的一份礼物》的演讲时说:"青蒿素是人类征服疟疾进程中的一小步,也是中国传统医药献给人类的一份礼物。"屠呦呦发现青蒿素,是从东晋时期葛洪所著《肘后备急方》中获得了启发。她发现书中记载了公元400年左右时青蒿被用来治疗间歇性发热(疟疾的一种症状)。屠呦呦在谈到关键的中医文献对她的启示时表示,当年自己面临研究困境时,又重新温习中医古籍,进一步思考东晋葛洪《肘后备急方》有关"青蒿一握,以水二升渍,绞取汁,尽服之"的截疟记载。这使她联想到提取过程可能需要避免高温,由此改用低沸点溶剂的提取方法。

In her speech titled "Artemisinin is a Gift from TCM to the World" delivered at Karolinska Institute in Sweden, Tu Youyou declared that "Artemisinin is a small step in the process of human conquest of malaria and a gift to mankind from Traditional Chinese Medicine." Her inspiration for the discovery of artemisinin came from the ancient medical book *Handbook of Prescriptions for Emergencies* compiled by Ge Hong of the Eastern Jin Dynasty. She found evidence in this book which claimed that *qinghao* (sweet wormwood) was used to tackle intermittent fevers (a symptom of malaria) around 400 A.D. As regards the cues from key TCM documents, she said in those days when she got into difficulties, she brushed up the Chinese ancient medical books again and further reflected the records in *Handbook of Prescriptions for Emergencies* compiled by Ge Hong, which gave detailed accounts of preventing malaria: "Take a handful of *qinghao* (artemisinin), soak them in two liters of water, wring out the juice and take it all." This reminded her that the high temperature caused by heating during extraction may need to be avoided and thus the problem was eased by switching to the lower boiling point by mimicking the original formula in the book.

关于青蒿入药,最早见于马王堆三号汉墓的帛书《五十二病方》,其后的《神农本草经》《补遗雷公炮制便览》《本草纲目》等典籍都有青蒿治病的记载。屠呦呦引用毛泽东主席的话呼吁:"'中国医药学是一个伟大的宝库,应当努力发掘,加以提高。'青蒿素正是从这一宝库中发掘出来的。"

The first evidence of artemisia annua used as medicine was found in the silk manuscripts of a Chinese medical book entitled *Recipes for 52 Kinds of Disorders* unearthed from the third Han Tomb at Mawangdui. Its application could also be found in other Chinese medical classics such as *Shennong's Classic of Materia Medica*, *Handbook of Addendum for Processing Drugs by Lei Gong*, *Compendium of Materia Medica*, etc. Tu quoted late Chairman Mao Zedong as saying that "More potential exploration and improvement for TCM should be carried out for it is a great treasure house." "It was precisely from such a great treasure house that *qinghao* (artemisinin) was discovered." she added.

据《中国疫病史鉴》记载,自西汉以来的2000多年里,中国先后发生过三百多次疫病,皆因中医药的有效预防和治疗,才控制住了疫情的蔓延。继2003年非典型性肺炎之后,2020年以来,中医药抗击新冠肺炎不仅在国内再次发挥了重要作用,而且其全球影响力也在不断扩大。在历次重大疫情面前,中医药焕发出它历久弥新的生命力。

As stated in *Historical References for Epidemic Diseases in China*, over the past 2,000 years since the Western Han Dynasty (206 B.C.-8 A.D.), more than 300 epidemic diseases unfolded in Chinese history. The spread of epidemic diseases were all under control due to the effective prevention and treatment of TCM. Since the outbreak of COVID-19, TCM not only plays a big health role in China's fight against the coronavirus but also expands its global presence amid COVID-19 fight after combating the deadly outbreak of Severe Acute Respiratory Syndrome (SARS) across China in 2003. In the face of all previous major epidemic diseases, TCM has always been shining with a striking tenacious vitality which is always new.

几千年来,中医药为中国人民治愈了无数的疾病,减轻了他们的痛苦,为世界健康开出"中国药方",为中华民族的繁衍和昌盛做出了巨大的贡献,也对世界文明产生了深远的影响。

For thousands of years, TCM, not only has cured numerous diseases and relieved sufferings for the Chinese people, but gives a "Chinese prescription", providing a healthy way of nursing the world. TCM has made a tremendous contribution to the reproduction and prosperity of the Chinese nation, also has produced far-reaching impact on the world civilization.

第二篇 中医基础理论

Section 2 Fundamental Theories of TCM

  中医学理论体系是以整体观念为指导思想,以辨证论治为诊治特点,以唯物论和辩证法思想、阴阳五行学说为哲学基础,以脏腑、经络、气血津液为生理、病理基础的独特的医学理论体系。中医基础理论是中医学理论体系的重要组成部分,是指导中医预防医学和临床医学的理论基础。

  TCM theoretical system is a unique theoretical system of medicine which stresses upholding the holistic view as the guiding ideology, treatment based on syndrome differentiation as the characteristic of diagnosis and treatment, materialism and dialectics, together with theory of yin-yang and the five elements as the philosophical basis, the viscera, meridians, qi, blood and body fluid as the physiological and pathological basis. The fundamental theories of TCM, which are key components of TCM theoretical system, serve as the theoretical base for preventive medicine and clinical medicine in TCM.

第一章　整体观念

"我们没有特效药,但是我们中医找到了解决方案,解决了问题。"为疫情防控做出重大贡献而获"人民英雄"国家荣誉称号的中医专家张伯礼在与国外分享防治新冠病毒经验时表示,身体生病了就像屋子里堆积的垃圾生了虫子,我们不去抓虫子,而是去清除垃圾堆,通过改善身体机能来实现健康的目的。这也是中医整体观念的胜利。

Chapter 1　Holistic View

"There is still no specific cure for novel coronavirus, but traditional Chinese medicine has already arrived at a health solution and ultimately solved the problem." said Zhang Boli, a TCM expert and a recipient of the "People's Hero" national honorary title for his outstanding contributions to the country's fight against the coronavirus pandemic (COVID-19). "A sick body is just like a garbage-piled room with bugs everywhere. Instead of bug-hunting, our priority is rightly to get rid of the garbage. TCM aims to reach the goal of health by means of improving functioning capabilities of the body. This is also a victory of TCM holistic approach." Zhang made the remarks when sharing with foreign countries the information and experience in the COVID-19 prevention and treatment.

中医理论建立在中国古代哲学思想的基础之上,整体论就是这样的哲学。在中医看来,人体本身是一个有机的整体,整体即事物的统一性和完整性。中医重视人体本身的统一性、完整性以及与自然界的相互关系。和西医不同,中医对人体有独到的理解,认为人体脏腑、器官、组织是整体的一部分,而人体的所有这些部分构成一个整体。整体是具有不同功能的各个部分的总和。因而构成人体的各个组成部分在生理上相互联系、相互协调;在功能上相互作用;在病理上则相互影响。机体整体性的形成,是以五脏为中心,配之以六腑,通过经络系统"内属于腑脏,外络于肢节"的作用实现的。人体某一局部区域内的病理变化往往与人体阴阳的盛衰有关。中医眼里的疾病,不只是某个局部器官组织的病变,而是病人整体机制出现了某种失衡。所以中医不会特意治疗人体某个局部区域的病变,而是把病人视为一个整体来诊断疾病,并提出相应的治疗方案,以期恢复身体的平衡。

The theory of TCM is based on ancient Chinese philosophical thoughts. The holism theory is such a philosophy. In TCM, human body is an organic whole. A holistic view means unity and integrity. TCM values the relationship between unity and integrity of the human body itself, as are the relationship between human and nature. Unlike western medical approach, TCM has a unique understanding of the human body. TCM philosophy holds that the micro-unit, such as viscera, organs and tissues, is part of the whole and all these parts of the body build a oneness. The whole is the total of its parts which possess different functions. The components of human body physiologically connect and coordinate with each other, functionally reinforce each other and pathologically affect each other. The unity of the body is realized through the dominant function of the heart with the aid of the six fu-organs together with the meridians which "pertain to the viscera in the interior and connect with the limbs and joints in the exterior". The pathological changes in certain part of the body are usually related to the conditions of yin and yang in the whole body. For a TCM practitioner, a disease is not merely pathology in certain local organ or tissue, but a loss of balance in the whole mechanism. Hence TCM practitioners will not treat a localized disorder specifically but will consider the body as a whole to diagnose the disorders and come up with corresponding therapeutic schedule so as to restore balance.

构成人体的各个组成部分相互影响、相互协调。正如《黄帝内经》所载："从阴引阳，从阳引阴，以右治左，以左治右"，再比如"病在上者下取之，病在下者高取之"，这些都是整体观治疗原则的体现。中医整体观认为人体本身是一个完整的体系。

Every part composing the body influences and coordinates with each other. Just as *Inner Canon of the Yellow Emperor* states that "Highly skilled acupuncture practitioners will always draw yang from yin, draw yin from yang; needle the acupoints located on the right side to treat disease on the left side and vice versa." For another example, "If the disease is in the upper part of the body, the acupoints located on the lower part of the body can be needled to receive treatment and the converse is also true." All these are reflections of holistic therapeutic principle. The holistic view of Chinese medicine believes that the human body itself is a complete system.

有这样一则笑话：从前有一位医生，自称擅长外科，军营里有位将士在战场上背部中箭，箭头深深扎进肉中，疼痛难耐，于是就请那位外科医生来施行手术。医生走近稍一察看，就掏出一把大剪刀，"咔嚓"一声，把露在外面的半截箭杆剪掉，便要离去。将士急忙拉住他说："箭头还扎在肉里面，怎么不取出来？"医生回答："这是内科的事情，与外科无关！"这位医生把局部和整体截然分开了，这和中医整体观正好背道而驰。

There was such a joke: Once upon a time there was a doctor who claimed to be good at surgery. A soldier in the barracks was shot in the back with an arrow on the battlefield. The arrow plunged deeply into his flesh and the pain was unbearable, so he asked the surgeon to perform the operation. The doctor approached and inspected it for a while, then took out a pair of big scissors, cutting off the half exposed arrow shaft. Then he was about to leave. The soldier hurriedly held him back and asked, "The arrowhead is still stuck in the flesh, why don't you take it out?" The doctor answered, "This is a matter of internal medicine, and has nothing to do with surgery!" This doctor completely separated the part from the whole which ran counter to the holistic view of Chinese medicine.

同时，就像人和社会的关系、人体的局部区域和整个身体的关系一样，人与自然有着密不可分的联系。自然界的运动和变化会直接或间接地影响人体，而人体也必然产生相应的生理或病理上的反应。中国人有句谚语叫"春捂秋冻，不生百病"，意思是说人与自然是一个整体，人的生活起居要顺应自然规律，这就是中医整体观的具体反映。

Simultaneously, TCM deems that the relationship between human and nature is an inseparable whole, as are the relationships between human and the society, and between the local areas and the whole body. The movement and changes in the natural world will directly or indirectly affect human body, and human body will inevitably produce physiological or pathological reflections accordingly. Just as an old Chinese proverb goes, "Wearing more in spring and less in autumn", which means that man and nature are an integrated whole and one's daily routine should conform to natural law. This is a specific reflection of the holistic view of TCM.

人既是自然的产物，又是自然的延伸和精华。人与自然服从宇宙同一法则即所谓的"宇宙之道"："人道"依存于"天道"，"天道"服务于"人道"。如此便形成了中医独特的整体观和辨证论治的核心价值。中医理论体系的两个基本特点就是整体观和辨证论治。

Human being is not only a product of nature, but also an extension and essence of nature. Both human being and nature are subject to the same law known as *dao* (law of the universe). *Tiandao* (law of nature) depends on *rendao* (law of human), and *rendao* (law of human) in its turn serves *tiandao* (law of nature). The interaction of both paves way to the core values of TCM which involve holistic view and treatment based on syndrome differentiation. The theoretical system of TCM is characterized by the following two essential characteristics: holistic view and treatment based on syndrome differentiation.

季节的变化，会直接或间接地影响人的身体，从而引起相应的生理或病理上的反应。如《黄帝内经·素问》所载："春夏养阳，秋冬养阴，以从其根。"在大自然气候变化的影响下，生物会有春生、夏长、长夏化、秋收、冬藏等适应性的变化。所以，整体观认为顺应自然，因循四时变化规律，与大自然和社会环境保持协调一致，对健康有着重要影响。正如《黄帝内经·灵枢》所载："天暑衣厚则腠理开，故汗出；天寒则腠理闭，气湿不行，水下留于膀胱，则为溺与气。"而且，整体观认为人的身心是一体的，强调身体和精神之间的相互协调与相互作用。中医认为身心整体的和谐是健康的基础。这种内外环境的统一性、机体自身整体性的思想，就是整体观的核心。

Seasonal changes may directly or indirectly influence the body, and accordingly cause physiological or pathological reactions. Just like *Plain Questions* states that "One should cultivate yang in spring and summer while nourish yin in autumn and winter so as to cement the health foundation." Under the influence of climate changes of nature, the living things on the earth will also change to adapt to environmental variation, such as sprouting in spring, growing in summer, alteration in late summer, ripeness in autumn and storage in winter. Therefore, a holistic view holds that it is important for health to follow the laws of nature, conform to seasonal changes and achieve harmony with nature and social environment. As *Spiritual Pivot* states that "The skin tends to excrete sweat as a result of the open muscular interstices when one puts on more clothes in summer, while body fluid will be held up in the bladder to form urine or to cause retention of urine as a result of the closed muscular interstices and detained dampness when the weather turns cold." Moreover, a holistic view holds that the mind and body are one, underlining the coordination and interactions of physical and mental factors. In TCM, the harmony of the body and soul is the basis for health. The idea of the unity of the internal and external environment, and the integrity of the body itself is the kernel core of the holistic view.

整体观源自中国古代"天人相应"的思想,在这一思想的指导下,疾病的诊治必须整体分析与调治。整体观贯穿在中医生理、病理、辨证、诊治等各个方面。

The holistic view originates from the ancient Chinese thought of "Correspondence between Man and Nature". Under the guidance of such an idea, TCM has remained a truly holistic approach to diagnosis and treatment in terms of analyzing and regulating the disease. A holistic view of health threads through all aspects of TCM, such as physiology, pathology, dialectics, diagnosis and treatment, etc.

第二章　辨证论治

相传有一次华佗碰到两个患头痛的病人,他们的症状完全一样。华佗诊脉以后,断定一位叫倪寻的病人应当服泻药,而另一位叫李延的病人则应服用发汗药。两人分别服了华佗开的药之后,头痛病都痊愈了。有人问华佗为什么对同样的病却要用不同的药来治疗,华佗解释说:"倪寻的病根在内部,所以要用泻药;李延的病则是受外邪侵袭,所以要用发汗药。"这则逸闻说明华佗灵活运用了中医辨证论治的原则。中医强调辨证,因为只有准确辨证,才能正确治疗。

Chapter 2　Treatment Based on Syndrome Differentiation

Legend had it that once Hua Tuo encountered two patients, both of whom suffered from headaches with the same symptoms. After feeling their pulses, Hua Tuo came to the conclusion that a purgative therapy would be a better option for the patient named Ni Xun, while a sudatory one would benefit the other patient named Li Yan. Both of them took their medicine respectively and made their recovery. When Hua Tuo was asked why different cures were adopted for the same disease, he put it this way, "Ni Xun's root of disease exists internally, and hence the purgative works. While sudatory is the right remedy for Li Yan for exogenous pathogenic factors invasion appeared to be the precise nature of his illness." This anecdote demonstrated that Hua Tuo had flexibly adopted the principles of TCM treatment based on syndrome differentiation. TCM emphasizes the differentiation of syndrome, because only when the syndrome is accurately differentiated can a proper treatment be made.

"辨证论治"这个概念出自东汉末年医学家张仲景所著《伤寒杂病论》,这部经典确立了辨证论治的原则，对后世临床实践具有非常重要的意义。所谓"辨证"，就是辨别、分析、总结疾病的证候。辨证包括八纲辨证、气血津液辨证、脏腑辨证、病因辨证、经络辨证、卫气营血辨证和三焦辨证。"论治"就是根据辨证的结果确立相应的治疗方法。辨证是论治的前提和依据；论治则是依据辨证治疗疾病的方法和手段。辨证论治是中医认识和治疗疾病的基本法则。

The concept "treatment based on syndrome differentiation" came from *Treatise on Febrile Diseases and Miscellaneous Illnesses* by a leading ancient Chinese medical scientist Zhang Zhongjing at the end of the Eastern Han Dynasty. This classic, which established the principle of treatment based on syndrome differentiation, was of great significance for the later clinical practice. The so-called "syndrome differentiation" is a matter of identifying, analyzing and summarizing symptoms of diseases. "Syndrome differentiation" involves differentiation of syndromes in accordance with the eight principle syndromes; with the state of *qi*, blood and body fluid; with the state of the *zang-fu* organs; with etiological analysis; with the meridian and collateral theory; with the defensive, *qi*, nutritive and blood systems and with triple energizer theory. "Treatment determination" indicates adopting corresponding therapeutic methods according to the results of syndrome differentiation, which is the prerequisite and basis for determining treatment. "Treatment determination" is exactly the methods and means to treat diseases in the light of syndrome differentiation. In TCM, treatment based on syndrome differentiation is the basic principle for disease perception and treatment.

关于辨证论治有很多逸闻趣事。相传有一次两个病人找张仲景治病，他们的症状相同，都是因为淋雨而导致重感冒，表现为头痛、咳嗽和鼻塞。张仲景切脉后给他们都开了麻黄汤来发汗退热。然而第二天，一位病人的亲属急匆匆地来告诉他，病人发汗了，但服药后头痛得更加厉害了。张仲景为他的错误诊断担心不已并去看望了另一位病人。让他感到欣慰的是，另外一位病人服药之后病情减轻了。张仲景百思不得其解：两位病人因为患同样的病服用了同样的药，但是效果大相径庭。他考虑再三，回想起一位病人脉弱并且腕上有汗，但是另一位病人腕上根本无汗。他想起来他忽略了两位病人的这点差别。发汗的病人服药之后出汗更多，因此变得愈加虚弱，病情加重。因此，他立即改变了治疗方法，重新为病人开了药方。最终，病人很快康复了。中医强调辨证论治，症状虽然相同，但引起疾病的原因不同，所以治疗方法也有所不同。

Numerous anecdotes attached to treatment based on syndrome differentiation came out as the wave of TCM surged. According to legend, once two patients who both had bad colds with the same symptoms of headache, cough and stuffy nose for being caught in a heavy rain came to him for cures. After feeling pulses for them, Zhang Zhongjing prescribed the same *mahuang* decoction for them to induce perspiration and bring down a fever. On the following day, however, a relative of one of patient came to Zhang Zhongjing hastily and told him that the patient sweated out, but the headache got worse after taking the medicine. Zhang Zhongjing worried about his error diagnosis and rushed to visit the other patient. To his relief, the other got much better after taking the medicine. Scratching his head, Zhang Zhongjing got very puzzled. The two patients took the same medicine due to the same disease, but the effects were quite different. He thought it over and recalled that one patient's pulse was weak with sweat on the wrist, but there was no sweat on the other's wrist at all. It occurred to him that he overlooked this difference between the two patients. The patient with sweat became weaker because he sweated out more after taking the medicine, and it made the disease get worse. Therefore, the search for another cure went on immediately. He prescribed medicine for the patient again and finally the patient recovered soon. TCM emphasizes treatment based on syndrome differentiation. Although the symptoms are the same, the treatment varies with the causes of the disease.

由此可见，中医诊治并非着眼于"病"的异同，而是着眼于"证"的异同。"同病异治，异病同治""证同治亦同，证异治亦异"就是辨证论治实质的体现。辨证论治是中医的灵魂。

It is readily apparent that the diagnosis and treatment of TCM centers around the "syndrome pattern" differentiation instead of "disease" differentiation. The tenet such as "treating the same disease with different therapies" "treating different diseases with the same therapy" "the same treatment for the same pattern and different treatments for different patterns" are all manifestations of the essence of treatment based on syndrome differentiation, which is the soul of TCM.

中医在其形成过程中受到了古代唯物论和辩证法思想的深刻影响。在中医发展的漫长过程中,辩证法贯穿其中。传统中医的精髓是治病需治本。辨证论治的核心就在于治病要抓住疾病的内在根本而非外显的症状。辨证和论治是诊治过程中两个相互联系、不可分割的方面,是理论和实践的结合。

During the process of its formation, TCM has been under the profound influence of ancient Chinese materialism and dialectics. In the long course of TCM's development, dialectics has been permeated in all aspects of TCM. At the heart of TCM is the principle that the root cause of disease, not its symptoms, is the essence of disease diagnosis and treatment. The core of treatment based on syndrome differentiation is to seize the internal causes instead of external manifestations of a disease. Differentiation of syndrome, coupled with treatment determination, serves as two interrelated and inseparable aspects in diagnosing and treating disease, embodying the combination of theory and practice.

第三章　取象比类

　　所谓"取象比类",又称"援物比类",是中国古代传统文化中特有的认知方法。比如《道德经》中所说的"上善若水",《黄帝内经·素问》中记载的"春脉如弦",这些就是用比喻的方式来说明事物的本质特征。取象比类是运用形象思维来比较被研究对象与已知对象在某些方面的相似或类同之处,以此来理解和巩固信息。用一个概念来阐释另一个概念有助于利用一个概念的本质特征来解释抽象的部分。往往一个恰当的比喻就可以令人茅塞顿开,把抽象复杂的东西讲明白,让人悟出深刻的道理。

Chapter 3　Drawing Analogies

　　Drawing analogies, also known as "analogy of related matters", is a unique cognitive method in ancient Chinese traditional culture. As stated in *Tao Te Ching*, "The highest good is like water." And in *Plain Questions*, it also has made mention of it, "The pulse in spring feels the way one rests his fingers on the taut or wiry strings of a musical instrument." That's how we explain the essential characters of things in a figurative way. Drawing analogies is a cognitive method that adopts thinking in images to compare something similar or in common between the research object and the known object so as to understand and cement information. Using one concept to illustrate another will aid capturing the essential features of such a concept to explain the abstract. In most cases, one may become enlightened all of a sudden through an appropriate analogy. Drawing analogies makes the abstract and complex things clear, enabling one to realize the profound truth.

　　人们为了变未知为已知,常把生疏的对象与熟悉的事物相比类,中医有很多基本知识都是借助这一方法衍生得来的。如自然界有风吹树倒的现象,故而中医认为人体四肢、头部不自主地摇动或人突然昏倒,均为风所致。取象比类是中医理论最基本的建构方法。

In order to change the unknown to the known, people always compare unfamiliar objects with familiar ones. In TCM, lots of the basic knowledge is generated by this method. For example, there is a phenomenon of wind blowing down trees in the natural world. TCM deems that the involuntary shaking of human limbs or head and a sudden faint are all caused by such wind. Drawing analogies is the most basic construction method of TCM theory.

中医运用五行学说,采用取象比类的方法,对人体的生理、病理现象以及与人类生活密切相关的自然界事物,按照其不同性质与功能,分别将其归类到金、木、水、火、土五行之中,借以阐述人体五脏六腑之间生理、病理方面的复杂联系,以及人体与外界之间的相互关系。例如,木有生长、升发、条达舒畅的特性,中医把性喜条达舒畅的肝脏归类到木;土有生化、承载、受纳的特性,中医把运化水谷精微,化生气血以养五脏的脾脏归类到土,这些都是采用取象比类的方法。

TCM applies the five elements theory to explore physiological and pathological phenomena of the human body, as well as things in nature which are closely related to human life, ascribing things to metal, wood, water, fire and earth in the light of their different properties and functions by drawing analogies. In this way, TCM expounds the complex links among the viscera of the human body physiologically and pathologically, and its correlations between human body itself and the outside world. In TCM, for instance, the liver belongs to the wood with central features of growing, ascending and developing freely, and thus the liver which prefers to grow freely is attributed to the category of wood. The spleen performs the functions of transforming and transporting food nutrients to all parts of the body, and transforming *qi* and blood to nourish the five-*zang* organs for it belongs to the earth, which has characteristics of generating, holding and receiving. All of these are reflections of drawing analogies.

有句俗语叫"吃什么补什么",譬如看到核桃仁与大脑形状相似,所以认为吃核桃能补脑,这也是人类运用取象比类的思维方法认识世界的体现。

As a popular folk adage goes, "You are what you eat." It is a common Chinese culinary belief that eating a certain similar part nourishes the corresponding part in the human body. People describe the walnut kernel as the brain for its resemblance in shape to the brain, based largely on the application of the thinking method—drawing analogies.

据明朝许浩所著《复斋日记》记载,元末明初医学家滑寿,精于医道。他给人治病,从不拘泥于方书,而是根据病情灵活用药,凡经他医治,无不显效。有一年秋天,姑苏城内有一些做官的人邀请滑寿同游虎丘山。有一富贵之家的孕妇难产,想把滑寿拉回去诊治,而同游的人却不让他走。这时滑寿走到台阶上,看到一片刚落下的梧桐叶,就拾起来交给来人说:"赶快回去把这片梧桐叶用水煎了让孕妇喝下。"还未入席宴饮,就有人来报孩子已经生下来了。大家都问滑寿这是出自什么药方,滑寿回答道:"以意度之,何方之有?凡妇女怀胎十个月还没有生产的,是气不足的缘故。桐叶得秋天肃降之气而坠落,我凭借这个道理,用桐叶催生,产妇气足了,哪里还有不顺利生产的道理呢?"

According to *Diaries of Fu Zhai* by Xu Hao in the Ming Dynasty, Hua Shou, a distinguished physician of the late Yuan and early Ming Dynasties, was skilled in the art of healing. He treated the patients flexibly according to their concrete conditions instead of confining himself within the medical formulary. His regular treatment of patients was invariably effective. In one autumn, some officials in Suzhou invited Hua Shou to visit Huqiu Mountain. It chanced that a pregnant woman from a rich family had a difficult birth and intended to get him back for a cure. His companions, however, did not let him go. At this time Hua Shou walked onto the stone steps and saw a freshly fallen *wutong* (Chinese parasol) leaf. Hua Shou picked up the leaf, handed it to the messenger and said, "Hurry back and decoct this leaf with water for the patient to drink." When news came that a baby was born, Hua Shou and his companions had not started their feast yet. Everyone was asking about this magic prescription. Hua Shou explained, "There aren't any magic prescription, all it takes is to draw analogies between these two. The reason why a pregnant woman fails to bear a baby after ten months is that there is a deficiency of *qi*. Leaves of *wutong* (Chinese parasol) fall off the trees in the autumn conforming to the descending *qi* of this season. This also applies to fallen *wutong* (Chinese parasol) leaf assisting delivery. How can a pregnant woman have no smooth and easy delivery if there is sufficient *qi*?"

滑寿用桐叶催生,就是以落叶禀金气而坠落,来类比孕妇气足而产子,这就是取象比类的具体体现。

The situation that Hua Shou used the fallen *wutong* leaf to assist unsmooth delivery was analogous to leaves of *wutong* falling off the trees due to the predominant descending *qi* in autumn. This can be the concrete embodiment of drawing analogies.

第四章 阴阳学说

清代曹雪芹所著《红楼梦》中,中医药文化俯拾即是。在第三十一回"撕扇子作千金一笑,因麒麟伏白首双星",史湘云和丫鬟翠缕话阴阳。

湘云道:"花草也是同人一样,气脉充足,长得就好。"翠缕把脸一扭,说道:"我不信这话。若说同人一样,我怎么不见头上又长出一个头来的人?"湘云听了,由不得一笑,说道:"我说你不用说话,你偏好说。这叫人怎么好答言?天地间都赋阴阳二气所生,或正或邪,或奇或怪,千变万化,都是阴阳顺逆。多少一生出来,人罕见的就奇,究竟理还是一样。"翠缕道:"这么说起来,从古至今,开天辟地,都是阴阳了?"湘云笑道:"糊涂东西,越说越放屁。什么'都是些阴阳'。难道还有个阴阳不成!阴阳两个字还只是一字,阳尽了就成阴,阴尽了就成阳。不是阴尽了又有个阳生出来,阳尽了又有个阴生出来。"翠缕道:"这糊涂死了我!什么是个阴阳,没影没形的。我只问姑娘,这阴阳是怎么个样儿?"湘云道:"阴阳可有什么样儿,不过是个气,器物赋了成形。比如天是阳,地就是阴;水是阴,火就是阳;日是阳,月就是阴。"翠缕听了,笑道:"是了,是了。我今儿可明白了。怪道人都管着日头叫'太阳'呢,算命的管着月亮叫什么'太阴星',就是这个理了。"湘云笑道:"阿弥陀佛!刚刚明白了。"翠缕道:"这些大东西有阴阳也罢了,难道那些蚊子、虼蚤、蠓虫儿、花儿、草儿、瓦片儿、砖头儿,也有阴阳不成?"湘云道:"怎么没有呢?比如那一个树叶儿,还分阴阳呢。那边向上朝阳的就是阳,这边背阴覆下的就是阴。"翠缕听了,点头笑道:"原来这样。我可明白了。只是咱们这手里的扇子怎么是阳,怎么是阴呢?"湘云道:"这边正面就是阳,那反面就为阴。"翠缕又点头笑了,还要找几件东西问,因想不起个什么来,猛低头就看见湘云宫绦上系的金麒麟,便提起来问道:"姑娘这个,难道也有阴阳?"湘云道:"走兽飞禽:雄为阳,雌为阴;牝为阴,牡为阳。怎么没有呢!"

Chapter 4 Theory of Yin-Yang

In the Chinese classic novel, *A Dream of Red Mansions* (one of the four ancient Chinese literature classics) by Cao Xueqin, TCM culture is plentifully available. In the 31st chapter of this ancient Chinese classic, Shi Xiangyun had one impressive exchange with her maid Cui Lv on yin and yang.

"Plants are like human beings," said Shi Xiangyun, "they grow well as long as the vitality generated by *qi* and blood is always sufficient."

"I don't believe this." Cui Lv gave a little twist of her head. "If they are alike, why can't I see a man growing out a new head on top of another?"

Shi Xiangyun could not repress a smile at this. "You'd better not make remarks about things that you don't know at all. Why must you do it that way? How can I shed some light for you? All things between heaven and earth stem from the interaction of yin and yang. It might be good or evil, strange or weird, ever-changing, but with all things we end up going for or against yin and yang. The same is true for some who were born with one-of-a-kind gifts."

Cui Lv responded, "In this light, all things can be attributed to yin and yang when heaven was separated from earth since ancient times?"

"You're talking like a salve to your paste-addled mind. You stupid thing." Shi Xiangyun said with a laugh. "How could there be so many yins and yangs? Yin and yang are one. The end of yang is the start of yin, and vice versa. It's not a case of whether the end of yin would generate another yang or not."

"I'm afraid you've lost me there," said Cui Lv, "what on earth are you talking about, Miss? Since yin and yang have neither form nor shape, how can I know their true features?"

"Yin and yang are nothing but *qi*. When they find a carrier, they give things their shapes. For example, heaven pertains to yang while earth belongs to yin; water to yin while fire to yang; the sun to yang while the moon to yin."

"Precisely!" Cui Lv smiled. "I've got it! No wonder people call the sun '*taiyang*', and fortune-tellers call the moon '*taiyinxing*'. That might be it."

"Amitabha! You are really into it now." Shi Xiangyun smiled. "That will be fine if those big things have yin and yang. Could it be that mosquitoes, fleas, midges, flowers, grass, tiles, and bricks also have yin and yang?" Cui Lv asked.

"They are of no exception. The leaf, for instance, has its yin and yang. The side facing the sun is yang and the reverse side is yin."

"Aha! That's it. I know what you're saying." Cui Lv nodded and smiled. "But what about the yin and yang in the fan I'm holding?"

"The front of the fan is yang and the back is yin."

Cui Lv nodded and smiled again. She could not help pursuing this matter, but she could not think of anything at that moment. Lowering her head fiercely, she saw the golden unicorn which her miss was wearing as a pendant.

"Does this also have yin and yang?" she asked.

"Sure enough! the birds and animals all have yin and yang. The male is yang and the female is yin."

这就是曹雪芹眼中的阴阳,世间万物,大到日月天地,小到花草飞虫,追根溯源,无不是因阴阳而起。
This was how Cao Xueqin saw the world in terms of yin and yang. In his eyes, everything in the world, as

large as the sun, the moon, the heaven, and the earth, or as small as the flowers, grass, and flying insects, all came from yin and yang if you were tracing to its source.

一、阴阳的基本概念

阴阳的概念,最早形成于夏商时期,战国时期阴阳理论的雏形已经初现。阴阳最早的文字记载见于殷商时期的甲骨文。在这些甲骨文中,有一些具有阴阳内涵的词语,如"阳日""晦月"等字样。《尚书》中曾有记载,山之南为阳,山之北为阴,这可以通过书法结构中的阴阳小篆书得到进一步证实。东汉许慎编撰的我国第一部字典《说文解字》曾载:"阴,暗也。水之南,山之北也。"春秋战国时期,中国古代哲学家和思想家老子在《道德经》中记载了"万物负阴而抱阳",认为万物都包含阴阳两个方面,阴与阳可通过气的运动变化达到完美的和谐状态,这标志着阴阳理论的初步形成。《周易》提出"一阴一阳之谓道",认为阴阳的相互作用是宇宙变化的根本规律,阴阳相合,万物生长。在天形成风、云、雷、雨等自然气象;在地则形成江湖河海、五岳山川等大地形体;在方位是东、南、西、北;在气候则为春、夏、秋、冬。阴阳观念最早应用到医学领域的记载见于《左传》,秦朝名医医和在为晋侯(晋国国君)诊病时,以阴阳解释疾病的病因。此后,《黄帝内经》系统阐述了阴阳学说,在这部经典中,阴阳学说贯穿始终。

1. Fundamental Concept of Yin-Yang

The concept of yin-yang could be said to date back to the Xia and Shang Dynasties, and the theory of yin-yang took shape during the Warring States Period. So far, the earliest written records of yin and yang in China appeared in oracle bone inscriptions during the Yin-Shang Period (1300 B.C. – 1046 B.C.), on which there were words carrying yin-yang connotations such as *yangri* (daytime sun) and *huiyue* (night moon), etc. In the classic *Book of*

Political and Historical Documents, yang was defined as south of a hill, whereas yin as north of a hill. This could be further confirmed by *xiaozhuan* (ancient form of Chinese writing) of yin and yang in calligraphic structure. In the *Shuo Wen Jie Zi*, China's first dictionary compiled by Xu Shen during the Eastern Han Dynasty, yin was defined as "Darkness, north of a hill and south of a river."

During the Warring States Period, ancient Chinese philosopher and thinker Laozi wrote in *Tao Te Ching*: "All things carry the yin at its back and yang in front", conveying the idea that everything had dual aspects of yin and yang. Through the motion and variation of qi, interactions between yin and yang could reach a perfect state. This also symbolized the embryo of yin-yang theory. According to *Books of Changes*, "Yin and yang make up the *dao* (law)", which held that the interaction of yin and yang was the fundamental law of changes of the universe. It was believed that the unity of yin and yang propelled the growth of everything on earth: meteorologically wind, cloud, thunder and rain; geographically river, lake, sea and mountain; spatially east, west, south and north; and seasonally spring, summer, autumn and winter. The earliest medical reference of yin and yang could be found in *Chronicle of Zuo*, according to this classic, when Duke Ping of Jin (the ruler of the state of Jin) got ill, Yi He, a famous doctor in the Qin Dynasty (221 B.C.-207 B.C.), was sent over to find a cure. Yin qi and yang qi were interpreted by Yi He for an explanation of the causes of diseases. After that, the yin-yang theory had been systematically elaborated in *Inner Canon of the Yellow Emperor*. In this classic, yin-yang theory threaded through the whole book.

正如中医典籍《黄帝内经》所载:"人生有形,不离阴阳。"自然界和宇宙千变万化,纵然错综复杂、扑朔迷离,究其根源,无不是阴阳相互作用的结果。"阴阳者,天地之道也,万物之纲纪,变化之父母,生杀之本始。"中医认为,阴阳的变化是世间万物变化的基本规律。

Just like TCM classics *Inner Canon of the Yellow Emperor* states that "Man has a physical shape which is inseparable from yin and yang." The ever-changing nature and the universe, despite their complex and eye-confusing nature, are all the result of the interaction between yin and yang if we search to the bottom of its intricacies. "Yin and yang are the law of heaven and earth, the principles of all things, the parents of all changes, and the origin of life and death." TCM believes that the change of yin and yang is the basic law of the world.

　　阴阳最初的含义甚为朴素,它来自中国古代哲学的概念。它指的是日光的向背,向日为阳,背日为阴。在后来的生活实践中,阴阳的含义逐渐引申、扩展,乃至被用来概括所有相互对立的两个方面。最初,阴代表月亮,阳代表太阳。这些概念逐渐扩展到阴代表夜晚,阳代表白昼;阴代表冬天,阳代表夏天;阴代表女性,阳代表男性。事实上,世间万物皆可从阴阳的角度来概括。古人开始意识到自然界所有的事物都有两个方面的特性,均可用阴阳加以解释,例如,天与地,白昼与黑夜,明亮与阴暗,运动与静止,方位的上下,升和降,出和入,热和冷等。前者属阳,后者属阴。关于阴阳这对矛盾范畴,最好的例子就是水火之间的关系。正如《黄帝内经·素问》有云:"水火者,阴阳之征兆也。"阳体现火的基本性质,那些自然界属火的,如热、运动、明亮、方位的上和外、兴奋和力量都属于阳;而阴则体现水的基本性质,那些自然界属水的,如冷、静止、阴暗、方位的下和里、颓丧和无力都属于阴。水寒凉润下,火炎热上升,故而水火可以作为阴阳的征兆。

　　The early connotations of yin and yang, which came from an ancient philosophical concept, were quite plain. The side facing the sun was yang and the reverse side was yin. In the course of later daily practice, yin and yang gradually extended and expanded to express all these dual and opposite qualities in the world. Originally, yin and yang represented the moon and the sun respectively. Gradually these terms extended to yin as night and yang as day; yin as winter and yang as summer; yin as female and yang as male. Actually, there was nothing which could not be viewed from the perspective of yin and yang. The ancients had become aware that all things in the natural world could be interpreted in the two conflicting ideas of yin and yang, for example, heaven and earth, day and night, brightness and dimness, motion and quiescence, upward and downward directions, ascending and descending, exiting and entering, heat and cold, etc. The former belongs to yang and the latter to yin in every pair mentioned above. The best example for the two opposite aspects of a contradiction is the relation between water and fire as described in *Plain Questions*, "Water and fire are the symbols of yin and yang." Yang manifests the basic nature of fire, such as heat, motion, brightness, upward and outward, excitement and power; while yin manifests the basic nature of water, such as coldness, stillness, dimness, downward and inward, depression and weakness. Water is cold, moistening and downward, while fire is blazing hot and upward, hence they can serve as signs of yin and yang respectively.

阴与黑色有关,代表着夜晚、寒冷、安静、被动、黑暗、内在、慢性疾病和女性;阳与白色有关,代表着白昼、温暖、运动、主动、明亮、外在、急性疾病和男性。每个人体内都有阴阳,但阴阳的比例各不相同。

Yin, which is associated with black, stands for night, coldness, quiescence, passivity, darkness, internality, chronic diseases and female; while yang, which has to do with white, is a symbol for day, warmness, motion, activity, brightness, externality, acute diseases and male. Yin and yang exist in each body but their respective proportion in each individual varies.

阴阳
Yin-Yang

二、阴阳理论的内容

中医认为,世界是阴阳相互作用的结果。阴阳的相互作用可简要概括为:阴阳对立、阴阳互根、阴阳消长和阴阳转化。

2. Content of Yin-Yang Theory

TCM believes that the world is the result of the interaction between yin and yang. The interaction between yin and yang can be distilled into four aspects: opposition of yin and yang, interdependence of yin and yang, wax-wane of yin and yang, transformation of yin and yang.

1. 阴阳对立

阴阳对立是指世间的一切事物和现象都存在着相互对立的两个方面。如天地、动静、升降、昼夜、热冷等。在每一组对立的组合中前者为阳,后者属阴。如以天地而言,天气轻清在上故属阳,地气重浊在下故属阴。正如《黄帝内经·素问》所载:"清阳为天,浊阴为地。"

（1）Opposition of Yin and Yang

Opposition of yin and yang means that all things and phenomena in the world have two opposite aspects known as yin and yang, such as heaven and earth, motion and quiescence, ascending and descending, day and night, heat and cold, etc. The former belongs to yang and the latter pertains to yin in every pair mentioned above which oppose each other. In terms of heaven and earth, the celestial qi is light and lucid, and thus pertains to yang; while the terrestrial qi is heavy and turbid, and therefore belongs to yin. In *Plain Questions*, it states that "The lucid yang ascends to form the heaven and the turbid yin descends to constitute the earth."

宇宙间一切事物的发生、发展和变化都是阴阳对立统一、矛盾运动的结果。人的生命活动过程就是人体中阴阳对立的双方在不断地矛盾运动中取得统一的过程。阴阳在相互对立、相互制约中实现统一。没有对立,就没有统一;没有制约,就没有互补。阴阳的动态平衡就是在这种相互对立和制约中实现的。中医用阴阳来阐释人和自然之间复杂的关系。自然界中天体的运动、四季的变化、晨昏的交替以及春生、夏长、秋收、冬藏无一不是阴阳对立统一关系的具体体现。

The occurrence, development and changes of all things in the universe are all the results of unity of opposites and contradictory movement between yin and yang. The course of life activity is a process in which yin and yang in the human body achieve unity through constant contradictory movement. Mutual opposition and restriction between yin and yang bring about unity. Without mutual opposition, there would be no unity; without mutual restriction, there would be no complementation. It is just through this kind of opposition and restriction that the dynamic balance of yin and yang can be realized. TCM adopts yin and yang to illustrate the complicated relationship between man and nature. In the natural world, the motions of celestial bodies, the variations of the four seasons, the alternations of days and nights as well as sprouting in spring, growing in summer, reaping in autumn and storing in winter are all concrete manifestations of the unity of opposites between yin and yang.

阴阳概念的前提是事物处在不断的运动变化之中。换句话说,没有任何事物是一成不变的,阴阳总是处在一种动态平衡之中。疾病的诊断治疗皆服从这一规律。正如《黄帝内经·素问》所载:"阴胜则阳病,阳胜则阴病。"《类经附翼》中也有类似的记载:"动极者镇之以静,阴亢者胜之以阳。"阴阳的对立统一处在不断的发展变化之中。故而《黄帝内经·素问》有云:"且夫阴阳者,有名而无形,故数之可十,离之可百,散之可千,推之可万。"

The prerequisite of the concept of yin and yang is that everything is in a constant state of change. In other words, nothing in the world remains the same. Yin and yang are always in a state of dynamic balance. No diagnosis and treatment of disease will exempt from this rule. As stated in *Plain Questions*, "Predomination of yin results in yang disease while predomination of yang leads to yin disease." A similar record can be found in *A supplement in Classification Classic*, "Those being too dynamic should be restrained by stillness, and those of yin-hyperactivity would be constrained by yang." The unity and opposition between yin and yang develop and change constantly. That is why it is said in *Plain Questions* that "Yin and yang own their names but no forms. Thus it can be extended from one to ten, ten to a hundred, a hundred to a thousand and a thousand to ten thousand."

2. 阴阳互根

阴阳互根是指阴阳既相互对立,又相互依存,任何一方都不能脱离另一方而单独存在。阳依存于阴,阴依赖于阳,每一方的存在都以另一方的存在为前提,故而"孤阴不生,孤阳不长"。

(2) Interdependence of Yin and Yang

Yin and yang are opposed to each other and at the same time depend on each other. One cannot exist without the other—that's the so-called interdependence of yin and yang. Without yin there would be no yang, and vice versa. Neither can exist in isolation. Therefore, "if only yang exists, there will be no birth; if only yin exists, there will be no growth".

中国古代哲学认为,万物的化生皆源于阴阳之间的相互作用。譬如,《荀子·礼论》认为"天地合而万物生,阴阳接而变化起"。宋朝哲学家周敦颐在《太极图说》中则提出"二气交感,化生万物"。

The generation and changes of all things on earth stem from the interaction between yin and yang in ancient Chinese philosophy. *Xunzi*: *Discourse on Ritual Principles*, for example, considers that "when heaven and earth integrate, everything is born; when yin and yang conjoin, changes will take place". During the Song Dynasty, in philosopher Zhou Dunyi's *On Taiji Diagram*, he wrote that "When yin *qi* and yang *qi* interact, all things are produced."

阴阳学说认为阴阳相互联系、相互依存,这种关系也反应在物质与功能的关系之中。物质属阴,功能属阳。没有无功能的物质,也没有无物质的功能。物质居于体内,功能表现于外。正如《黄帝内经·素问》所载:"阴在内,阳之守也。阳在外,阴之使也。"整个宇宙都处在阴阳的相互作用和交替之中。

Yin-yang theory deems that yin and yang are interconnected and interdependent. Such relationship is also reflected in the relationship between substance and function. Substance pertains to yin and function belongs to yang. There is no substance without function and no function without substance. Substance resides in the body, while function manifests outside. As is stated in *Plain Questions*, "Yin remains inside to guard yang while yang stays outside to protect yin." The entire universe is in the interaction and alternation of yin and yang.

3. 阴阳消长

阴阳消长是宇宙的基本规律。阴阳消长是指阴阳双方并非处于静止不变的状态,而是始终处于此盛彼衰、此增彼减的运动变化之中。其消长规律为阴消则阳长,阳消则阴长。阴阳相互制约的过程就是相互消长的过程。倘若阴阳失衡,疾病就会产生。

(3) Wax-Wane of Yin and Yang

The waxing-waning of yin and yang is the basic law in the universe. The wax-wane of yin and yang is not in a state of stillness, but in a state of dynamic change, usually manifesting as "yin wane with yang wax" "yang wane with yin wax" "yin increase with yang decrease" and "yang increase with yin decrease". Waning of yin will lead to the waxing of yang and vice versa—this makes the law. The process of mutual restriction between yin and yang is the course of waxing and waning between yin and yang. If the balance of yin and yang is broken, disease will consequently occur.

四季和气候的变化便是阴阳消长的具体体现。冬去春来,天气变暖;春尽夏至,天气渐热,这个过程就是所谓的"阴消则阳长"。反之,从夏到秋,天气变凉,从秋至冬,天气转冷,这个过程就是所谓的"阴盛则阳衰"。

The seasonal and climatic changes are concrete manifestations of waxing-waning of yin and yang. The weather gets warmer from winter to spring, and hotter from spring to summer. This process is the so-called "yin wane with yang wax". Conversely, the weather gets cooler from summer to autumn, and colder from autumn to winter. This process is the so-called "yin wax with yang wane".

当阳气过盛时，古人认为用音乐可以调节阴阳平衡。据《吕氏春秋·仲夏纪·古乐》记载，昔日朱襄氏一统天下之时，经常刮风，使得阳气蓄积过多，万物凋零，果实不成，故而朱襄氏让名叫"士达"的臣子弹奏五弦瑟来招阴气，以安定众生。

The ancients conceived that music could regulate the balance of yin and yang when there was excessive yang *qi*. According to *Spring and Autumn Annals of Lv Buwei*, in former days the land came under Zhuxiangshi's sway. Yang *qi* prevailed at that time for it was often windy. All things were dying and the fruits were visibly withered. Hence Zhuxiangshi ordered his minister named "Shi Da" to play the five-stringed plucked instrument to invite yin *qi* and soothe all living creatures.

而当阴气过盛时，古人就舞以导滞，疏散过多的阴气。相传尧的时代，人们就知道舞蹈能促进气的流动。据《吕氏春秋·仲夏纪·古乐》记载："昔陶唐氏之始，阴多滞伏而湛积，水道壅塞，不行其原，民气郁阏而滞著，筋骨瑟缩不达，故作为舞以宣导之。"这段记载不仅告诉我们古人追求阴阳平衡，而且舞蹈的出现和医学亦有渊源。

While when there was excessive yin *qi*, the ancient people would disperse stagnation by dancing so as to disperse the superfluous yin *qi*. In the times of Yao, people had already realized that dancing could promote the flow of *qi*. According to *Spring and Autumn Annals of Lv Buwei*, "During the early years of Taotangshi's reign, yin *qi* between heaven and earth tended to stagnate latently and accumulate gradually. Thus the water passages were blocked up and flows stopped in their original places. Yin *qi* thickened and was suppressed within the body. Muscles and bones therefore cowered and shrank, and then failed to extend properly. Hence dancing was created accordingly to disperse the stagnation and remove the obstruction." This record not only provided a glimpse into the ancients' pursuit of yin-yang balance, but showed that the first appearance of dancing was associated with medicine.

4. 阴阳转化

《老子》中有一句名言:"祸兮,福之所倚;福兮,祸之所伏。"老子认为祸福可以相互转化。同样,阴阳双方在一定条件下也可以互相转化。一方面,阴或阳会转化到它相反的一面,阴可以转化为阳,阳也可以转化为阴;另一方面,任何事物都可以被无限地分为阴阳两个方面。

(4) Transformation of Yin-Yang

As an ancient Chinese saying in *Laozi* goes, "Behind every good fortune lurks a bad fortune; behind every bad fortune rests a good fortune." Laozi believes that good fortune and bad fortune can be converted to one another. Similarly, under certain conditions, yin or yang may transform into its opposite side. On one hand, yin may be transformed into yang and vice versa. On the other hand, anything in the world can be divided into yin and yang infinitely.

阴阳转化的一个特点是这个过程并非是静止不变的。譬如山坡,白天阳光普照的一面是阳中寓阳,而背向阳光的一面则是阳中藏阴。到了夜晚,月光洒向之处则是阴中寓阳,而背向月光的一面则是阴中藏阴。正如《黄帝内经·素问》所载:"阴中有阴,阳中有阳。平旦至日中,天之阳,阳中之阳也;日中至黄昏,天之阳,阳中之阴也;合夜至鸡鸣,天之阴,阴中之阴也;鸡鸣至平旦,天之阴,阴中之阳也。"阴极必然生阳,一个最常见的说法就是"黎明之前是最黑暗的时候",反之亦然。

A characteristic of yin-yang transformation is that this process is not static but dynamic. Take a hillside as an example, during the day the sunlit side of the hill is yang within yang, while the shaded side is yin within yang. Conversely, at night the moonlit side of the hill is yang within yin, while the dark side of the hill is yin within yin. As stated in *Plain Questions*, "There is yin within yin and yang within yang. From dawn till noon, there is yang within yang for yang is predominant in the heaven, from noon till dusk yin within yang, from dusk till midnight yin within yin, and from midnight till dawn yang within yin." Excessive yin will definitely generate yang. An example of this can ben seen in the popular expression: "The darkest hour is right before the dawn." Naturally, the opposite is also true.

《黄帝内经·素问》中记载的"重阴必阳,重阳必阴""寒极生热,热极生寒"就是物极必反的道理。从病理上来看,阴证可以转化为阳证,反之亦然。

Records from *Plain Questions* indicate that "extreme yin turns into yang, and extreme yang turns into yin" "extreme cold brings on heat, and extreme heat brings on cold". That is why it is said that things will develop in the opposite direction when they go extreme. Pathologically, yin syndromes can be transformed into yang ones, and vice versa.

如果说阴阳的消长是量变的过程,那么阴阳的转化就是质变的过程。譬如,天气属阳,天气之所以下降而不上升,在于其中含有阴气,当阴气积聚到一定程度则会化为雨水;反之,地气属阴,地气之所以上升而不下降,在于其中含有阳气,当阳气积聚到一定程度则会升腾为云。故而《黄帝内经·素问》有云:"地气上为云,天气下为雨。雨出地气,云出天气。"

If the waxing-waning of yin and yang is a quantitative process, then the yin-yang transformation is a qualitative process. For example, the heaven *qi* belongs to yang. The reason why heaven *qi* has a tendency of falling downward instead of rising up is that heaven *qi* contains yin *qi*. When yin *qi* accumulates to a certain degree, it will drop in the form of rain. Conversely, earth *qi* pertains to yin. The reason why earth *qi* has a tendency of rising up instead of falling downward is that earth *qi* contains yang *qi*. When yang *qi* accumulates to a certain degree, it will rise to form clouds. Hence *Plain Questions* states that "The earth *qi* ascends to form clouds and the heaven *qi* descends to produce rain."

三、阴阳学说在中医中的应用

阴阳学说是构建中医理论的基石，它贯穿在中医理论体系的各个方面，用以阐释人与自然的关系、人体的生理功能及病理变化，指导临床诊断与治疗。

3. Application of Yin-Yang Theory in TCM

Considered a cornerstone of TCM theory, yin-yang theory permeates through all aspects of TCM's theoretical system, illustrating the relationship between man and nature, physiological function and pathological changes of the human body, and guiding clinical diagnosis and treatment.

中医典籍《黄帝内经》认为："从阴阳则生，逆之则死，从之则治，逆之则乱。反顺为逆，是谓内格。是故圣人不治已病治未病，不治已乱治未乱，此之谓也。夫病已成而后药之，乱已成而后治之，譬犹渴而穿井，斗而铸锥，不亦晚乎？"此段论述，可以说是阴阳学说在医学上的应用。中医典籍中类似的表述还有"阴阳交感""阴阳互根""孤阳不生""孤阴不长""重阴必阳""重阳必阴"等。中国文化寻求阴阳之间的平衡，认为唯此才能达到和谐。中医的阴阳哲学蕴含着无穷的智慧。

Inner Canon of the Yellow Emperor states that "One will be alive if he follows the principle of yin and yang, otherwise he will perish. Those who conform to the principle will be cured while those who prefer the other way might end up as a worsening case. Resistance instead of obedience to the yin-yang principle means killing oneself from within. That is the reason why a saint gives priority to prevention rather than cures. One takes precautions to nip the first signs of disease in the bud rather than wait until the disease has become a reality. Providing treatment after catching an illness, which can be comparable to digging a well after feeling thirsty or forging an ironclad shield after the breakout of war, is therefore too late." What this excerpt expounds is actually the application of yin-yang theory. Similar quotes from TCM classics are "interaction of yin and yang" "mutual rooting of yin and yang" "solitary yang failing to grow, solitary yin failing to increase" "extreme yin turning into yang, extreme yang turning into yin" and so on. Chinese culture seeks a balance between yin and yang. Only in this way can harmony be achieved. Embedded in yin-yang philosophy is infinite wisdom.

1. 阐释人体的组织结构

中医用阴阳理论来阐释人体器官组织复杂的关系。人体内为阴，外为阳；腹为阴，背为阳；脏腑之中，脏为阴，腑为阳；肝、心、脾、肺、肾五脏皆为阴；胆、胃、大肠、小肠、膀胱、三焦六腑皆为阳。故背为阳，阳中之阳，心也；背为阳，阳中之阴，肺也；腹为阴，阴中之阴，肾也；腹为阴，阴中之阳，肝也；腹为阴，阴中之至阴，脾也。

(1) Expounding Organic Structure of Human Body

TCM applies yin-yang theory to elucidate the complicated relationship of the body's organs and tissues. In terms of yin and yang, the interior of the body is yin and the exterior is yang. When speaking of yin and yang in the body, the abdomen is yin and the back is yang. When it comes to yin and yang of the *zang-fu* organs in the body, the *zang*-organs are yin and the *fu*-organs are yang. The five-*zang* organs—liver, heart, spleen, lung and kidney, are all yin; while the six-*fu* organs—gallbladder, stomach, large intestines, small intestines, urinary bladder and triple energizer, are all yang. The back is yang and the yang within the yang is the heart; the back is yang and the yin within the yang is the lung; the abdomen is yin and the yin within the yin is the kidney; the abdomen is yin and the yang within the yin is the liver; the abdomen is yin and the extreme yin within the yin is the spleen.

2. 阐释人体的生理功能

中医认为,阴阳平衡是维持人体正常活动的基础。反之,如果阴阳关系紊乱,则会导致疾病。故而《黄帝内经·素问》有载:"阴平阳秘,精神乃治;阴阳离决,精气乃绝。"

(2) Expounding Physiological Functions of Human Body

TCM believes that the balance of yin and yang serves as the basis to maintain the normal activities of human body. If such a balance is disturbed, disease will naturally occur. That is why it is recorded in *Plain Questions* that "The balance between yin and yang maintains full vitality; while the disintegration of yin and yang exhausts the essence and *qi*."

中医认为,人体的所有结构组织都是有机联系、不可分割的。以功能和物质的关系为例,人体的生理活动有赖于物质,没有物质,人体的生理活动无以为继,功能活动将无法实施。反之,功能活动又是人体物质生成的驱动力,没有功能活动,物质的新陈代谢将无法进行。如果功能与物质之间的关系失常,生命活动就会受到损害,从而导致阴阳分离、精气衰竭,甚至危及生命。

TCM holds that all the structures and tissues in the human body are organically connected and inseparable. Take the relationship between function and substance for example, physiological activities of the body depend on substance. Without substance, there would be no sustentation for the functional activities, the functional activities will have no way to be performed. Conversely, the functional activities are the driving force for the production of substance in the body. Without functional activities, the metabolism of the substance will be impossible. When the relationship between substances and functions gets abnormal, life activities will be broken, thus bringing about dissociation of yin and yang, depletion of the essence, and even an end of life.

3. 阐释人体的病理变化

中医运用阴阳理论来阐释人体的病理变化,指导临床诊断与治疗。从病理上来说,中医认为阴阳失衡是基本的发病机理之一。阴阳平衡才能维持人体正常的生理活动,如果阴阳失衡,疾病就会产生。

(3) Expounding the Pathological Changes of Human Body

Targeting at guiding clinical diagnosis and treatment, TCM applies yin-yang theory to expound pathological changes of human body. Pathologically, TCM considers that the imbalance between yin and yang is one of the basic pathogenesis of the disease. A balance of the yin and yang serves as the basis to maintain the normal activities of human body. If such a balance is disturbed, the diseases will arise.

中医认为,世界是阴阳二气相互作用的结果。倘若阴阳不能相互为用而是相互分离,人的生命也就终止了。阴阳的协调平衡是健康的表现。人体阴阳的任何一方虚损到一定程度,必然会导致另一方的不足。这种关系反映在生理上即为相互协调,反映在病理上即为相互影响。

TCM holds that the world is the result of the interaction of yin qi and yang qi. The separation of yin and yang instead of working for each other will lead to an end of life. The balance and harmony of yin and yang are the signs of good health. If the debility of yin or yang in the body develops to a certain degree, it will inevitably leads to insufficiency of the other side. A reflection of such an interaction manifests as intercoordination in physiology and as mutual interplay in pathology.

从病理上看,中医认为阴阳失衡是基本的发病机理之一。疾病的产生和发展与正气、邪气有关。正气和邪气的本质则依据阴阳的本质而定。正气和邪气之间的相互作用和相互斗争可以借由阴阳之间的关系来阐释。无论疾病的病理特征如何千变万化,都不外乎阴阳的偏盛偏衰。不管病理变化如何复杂,都可以通过阴阳的盛衰来分析总结。

Pathologically, TCM holds that the imbalance between yin and yang is one of the basic pathogenesis of the disease. The occurrence and development of disease are related to the healthy *qi* and pathogenic evil *qi*. The nature of both healthy *qi* and pathogenic evil *qi* can be classified according to the nature of yin and yang. The interaction and struggle between them can be explained in the light of the relations between yin and yang. No matter how ever-changing the pathogenic features of diseases are, they all can be attributed to the predominance or decline of yin and yang. No matter how complicated the pathological changes may be, they all can be analyzed and generalized as relative predominance or relative decline of yin and yang.

4. 指导临床诊断和治疗

由于疾病发生、发展的根本原因是阴阳失调,因此不管临床症状多么复杂和多变,都能用阴阳学说来阐释。《黄帝内经》中就有诸多相关记载:"阴胜则阳病,阳胜则阴病。阳胜则热,阴胜则寒。""重寒则热,重热则寒。""重阴必阳,重阳必阴。""阳虚则外寒,阴虚则内热。"对于中医而言,疾病诊断的关键在于通过阴阳学说识别病症以及关于阴阳失衡的诊断。

(4) Guiding Clinical Diagnosis and Treatment

Imbalance between yin and yang is the root cause for the onset and development of disease. Therefore, all clinical manifestations, no matter how complicated and changeable, can be elucidated by this theory. *Inner Canon of the Yellow Emperor* aims to give such a voice to Chinese doctors: "Predominance of yin leads to the disease of yang and predominance of yang results in the disease of yin; predominance of yang gives rise to heat syndrome and predominance of yin brings on cold syndrome." Relevent quotations from this classic are "extreme cold leading to heat and extreme heat resulting in cold" "extreme yin turning into yang and extreme yang changing into yin" "yang deficiency leading to exterior cold and yin deficiency bringing on interior heat". For a TCM practitioner, the kernel core of disease diagnosis lies in the identification of symptoms in terms of yin-yang and the diagnosis of yin-yang imbalances in TCM.

在诊断中,所有疾病皆可依据临床表现归纳为阴证或阳证。故《黄帝内经·素问》有云:"善诊者,察色按脉,先别阴阳。"如果阳虚,就无法抵御疾病入侵;如果阴虚,就无法为人体提供足够的支持和营养。阴虚势必导致阳虚,反之亦然。阴阳不仅互生而且互相转化。"夫邪之生也,或生于阴,或生于阳。其生于阳者,得之风雨寒暑;其生于阴者,得之饮食居处,阴阳喜怒。"一般来讲,符合阴的属性的证候称为阴证,如里证、寒证、虚证等;符合阳的属性的证候称为阳证,如表证、热证、实证等。

In diagnosis, all diseases can be boiled down to either yin syndrome or yang syndrome according to clinical manifestations. Therefore, it is recorded in *Plain Questions* that "Highly-skilled diagnosticians inspect complexion and feel pulse to differentiate yin from yang first." Deficiency of yang will fail to ward off the invasion of disease. Deficiency of yin will fail to provide enough support and nourishment for the body. Deficiency of yin will definitely result in deficiency of yang and vice versa. Yin and yang not only generate each other but also transform themselves into each other. "The occurence of pathogenic evil factors comes either from yin or yang. When it comes from yang, it stems from the attack of wind, rain, cold and summer-heat; when it comes from yin, it results from improper diet, living conditions and emotional changes." Generally speaking, syndromes pertaining to yin can be defined as yin syndromes, such as interior syndrome, cold syndrome and deficiency syndrome. Conversely, syndromes belonging to yang can be regarded as yang syndromes, such as exterior syndrome, heat syndrome and excess syndrome, etc.

在中医看来,阴阳学说可以被用来确立临床诊断和治疗原则,概括药物的性能、味道和功效,从而为临床用药提供理论依据。就药性而言,寒性者属阴,热性者属阳;就药味而言,酸、苦、咸属阴,辛、甜、淡属阳;就功效而言,收敛、沉降者为阴,发散、升浮者为阳。

In TCM, yin-yang theory is adopted not only for establishing clinical diagnostic and therapeutic principles but also for generalizing the property, flavor and efficacy of medicine so as to provide a theoretical basis for clinical practice. In terms of the medicinal properties, those with cold and cool nature pertain to yin, and those with hot and warm nature belong to yang. As to the flavor of medicine, those that are sour, bitter and salty in taste belong to yin and those that are acrid, sweet and bland in taste pertain to yang. Concerning the medicinal efficacy, those with astringent, descending and sinking function belong to yin, while those with dispersing, ascending and floating function pertain to yang.

总之,中医治疗疾病,就是根据病征的阴阳偏盛或偏衰来确定治疗原则,再结合药物的阴阳属性,选择相应的药物,使阴阳恢复平衡,从而治愈疾病。

On the whole, the therapeutic principle in TCM hinges on exuberance or debilitation of yin or yang. A combination with yin and yang properties of the medicine and a corresponding selection of proper medicine aid to restore the balance of yin and yang. This is how diseases are treated.

第五章　五行学说

一、五行学说的起源

五行最早被称为"五材"。据《左传》记载:"天生五材,民并用之,废一不可。"作为哲学概念,五行首次被明确记载的文章出自《尚书·洪范》。"五行:一曰水,二曰火,三曰木,四曰金,五曰土。水曰润下,火曰炎上,木曰曲直,金曰从革,土爱稼穑。润下作咸,炎上作苦,曲直作酸,从革作辛,稼穑作甘。"《尚书·洪范》的记载是对五行特性的经典概括。木、火、土、金、水在人类日常生产和生活中不可或缺,正如《尚书正义》所载:"水火者,百姓之所饮食也;金木者,百姓之所兴作也;土者,万物之所资生也,是为人用。"

Chapter 5　Theory of the Five Elements

1. Origin of the Five Elements Theory

The five elements, originally known as "five materials", are recorded in *Chronicle of Zuo* which states that "Nature produces five kinds of materials and the masses rely upon all these to live. None of them can be dispensed with". As a philosophical concept, the five elements are explicitly documented, for the first time, in another renowned ancient Chinese classic *Book of Political and Historical Documents*. According to this classic, "The five elements unveil themselves as water, fire, wood, metal, and earth. Water moistens and flows downward; fire burns and flares up; wood bends and stands straight; metal takes shape based on change and transformation, and earth supports sowing and reaping. The moistening and downward flowing water generates salty flavor; the flaming upward fire produces bitter flavor; the intertwined and upright wood develops sour flavor; the changing and reforming metal makes pungent flavor; and all grains, produced by earth, creates sweet flavor." *Book of Political and Historical Documents* provides a classic sum up for the characteristics of the five elements. Wood, fire, earth, metal, and water are indispensable part of daily life and production. Records of the five elements in *Revelation to the Book of History* unfold that "Water and fire are used for food and drink; metal and wood serve as construction and manufacture; and earth is responsible for the production of all things for people to use."

二、五行学说的基本概念

作为中医理论的基石之一,五行学说认为宇宙万物的属性都与木、火、土、金、水这五行相对应。五行学说主要用以分析各种事物的五行属性,也是研究事物之间相互联系的基本法则。中国古代劳动人民在长期的生活和实践中,认识到五行受日月和木、火、土、金、水五星的直接影响。后来,人们把木、火、土、金、水的属性加以抽象概括和延伸拓展,用来说明整个世界,并认为木、火、土、金、水既具有相互滋生、相互制约的关系,又处于不断运动变化之中,五行学说就此形成。五行学说也属于中国古代哲学范畴,是以木、火、土、金、水的特性来认识世界、解释世界和探求自然规律的一种宇宙观和方法论。

2. The Fundamental Concept of the Five Elements Theory

As one of the bedrocks of TCM, the five elements theory holds that everything in the universe corresponds to wood, fire, earth, metal and water. The five elements theory is used mainly in analyzing the properties of the five elements and exploring the basic law of the interrelation between things. Over thousands of years of life and practice, ancient Chinese people came to realize that yin-yang and the five elements were directly affected by the sun, the moon, and the five stars. People later abstracted and extended the properties of these five elements to elucidate the whole world, portraying the mutual generation and mutual restriction of these five elements. They also held that these five elements were in a state of constant move and change. Hence the theory of five elements took shape. The five elements theory, which is believed to be the cosmology and methodology for understanding and explaining the world based on the characteristics of five elements as well as exploring the natural law, falls into the category of ancient Chinese philosophy.

五行学说体现了唯物主义和辩证法的观点。与阴阳学说一样，五行学说亦成为中医学独特理论体系的组成部分。在古代，这一理论被应用于医学领域，极大地影响了中医理论体系的建立和发展，至今仍对临床医学实践起着指导作用。

The theory of five elements reflects a primitive view of materialism and dialectics. Like yin-yang theory, it has become a component of the unique theoretical system of TCM. In ancient times, this theory was applied to the field of medicine, thus dramatically affecting the establishment and development of the theoretical system of TCM. The theory of five elements has been playing a directive role in clinical medical practice up till now.

三、五行学说的基本内容

1. 五行的特性

根据五行理论，自然界的任何事物都是依据五行属性归类的。木的特性被概括为"木曰曲直"，故而凡具有生长、升发、条达舒畅特性的事物，均归属木；火的特性被概括为"火曰炎上"，故而凡具有温热、升腾特性的事物,均归属火;土的特性被概括为"土曰稼穑",故而凡具有生化、承载、受纳特性的事物,均归属土;金的特性被概括为"金曰从革",故而凡具有清洁、肃降、收敛等特性的事物,均归属金;水的特性被概括为"水曰润下",故而凡具有寒凉、滋润、向下运行特性的事物,均归属水。

3. The Basic Contents of the Five Elements Theory

(1) Characteristics of the Five Elements

According to the five elements theory, everything in nature is attributed to one of the five elements. Wood is characterized by "bending and standing straight", hence anything with characteristics of growing, ascending and developing freely is attributed to the category of wood. Fire is characterized by "burning and flaring up", hence anything with characteristics of warming and rising is attributed to the category of fire. Earth is characterized by "supporting sowing and reaping", hence anything with characteristics of generating, bearing, and receiving is attributed to the category of earth. Metal is characterized by "changing and reforming", hence anything with characteristics of purifying, descending and astringing is attributed to the category of metal. Water is characterized by "moistening and downward flowing", hence anything with the characteristics of cooling, moistening and moving downward is attributed to the category of water.

2. 五行的属性

中医认为五行中每一行都与人体内相应的器官有关。木与肝、胆有关;火与心、小肠有关;土与脾、胃有关;金与肺、大肠有关;水与肾、膀胱有关。

(2) Properties of the Five Elements

In TCM, each of the five elements is associated with a corresponding organ in the human body. Wood has to do with liver and gallbladder; fire with heart and small intestine; earth with spleen and stomach; metal with lung and large intestine; and water with kidney and urinary bladder.

肝主升而归属木；心阳主温煦而归属火；脾主运化而归属土；肺主肃降而归属金；肾主水而归属水。

Liver governs ascending and belongs to wood; heart yang governs warming and belongs to fire; spleen governs transportation and transformation and belongs to earth; lung governs purification and descending and belongs to metal; kidney governs water and belongs to water.

3. 五行之间的相互关系
自然界和人体内的五行相互作用。五行之间的相互关系主要有相生、相克、相乘、相侮以及母子关系等。
(3) Correlations among the Five Elements

The five elements interact with each other in the nature as well as in the human body. The correlations among the five elements are mainly characterized by inter-generation, inter-restriction, subjugation (over-restriction), counter-restriction, together with mutual interaction between mother-organ and child organ.

(1) 相生
五行相生，是指木、火、土、金、水之间存在着依次相互滋生、助长和促进的关系。五行之间依次滋生的次序是：木生火、火生土、土生金、金生水、水生木，木又复生火。
① Inter-Generation

The inter-generation of the five elements means that wood, fire, earth, metal, and water generate, bolster and promote each other. The five elements follow such an orderly productive cycle: Wood generates fire, fire generates earth, earth generates metal, metal generates water, and water in turn generates wood. Then wood kindles a fire again.

木为生火提供燃料,火燃尽,残留的灰烬归于土,为生物的繁衍提供了肥沃的土壤(营养)。土中蕴藏着各种矿物质和金属,冰冷的金属表面遇冷又会凝结出水珠。无水滋润,木难以成长,雨水使得植物在春天萌芽,浇水灌溉后,种子可以长成树木,从而完成五行的循环。

Wood provides fuel to create fire. Earth is produced from the ash left after such a fire, providing enriched soil (nourishment) for living things to flourish. From the earth come the metal and minerals. The cold metal surfaces cause water to condense. Without water there can be no growth, so the rain facilitates plants to sprout in the spring. When a seed is given water, it can grow into a tree (wood). Hence the cycle of the five elements is completed.

五行之间彼此动态相连,周而复始,循环不息。对于五行中的任何一行来说,都存在着"生我"和"我生"的关系。每一行既是"我生"之"子",又是"生我"之"母"。这种五行关系被称为"母子关系"。以木为例,木生火,所以木为火之母;而水又生木,故而木又为水之子。

The five elements are dynamically connected to each other, recurring in an everlasting cycle. Each of the five elements is marked by such relations as "being generated" and "generating". Each element is the "child" of the element that generates it and the "mother" of the one it generates. This relationship of the five elements is known as the "mother-child" relationship. Take wood for example, since wood generates fire, it is the mother of fire; wood is generated by water, hence it is the child of water.

(2) 相克

五行相克是指五行之间的相互克制和约束。五行相克的次序是:木克土、土克水、水克火、火克金、金克木。在这个循环相克的次序中,对于五行中的任何一行来说,都存在着"克我"和"我克"的关系。例如,金克木,木又克土。水能制火,火又能锻造金属。坚硬的金属可用于制木,而若无木的制约,土将坍塌。若无土的约束,水将流至最低处。五行相生相克,以此维持五行之间的平衡。

② Inter-Restriction

Inter-restriction implies bringing under control or restraint among the five elements. A controlling and restriction cycle of the five elements goes like this: Wood restricts earth, earth restricts water, water restricts fire, fire restricts metal and metal restricts wood. In this circular order, each of the five elements is marked by "being restricted" and "restricting". For example, metal restricts wood, and wood restricts earth. Water will keep fire under control and fire forges metal. The hardness of metal is expected to tame wood. Without the control of wood, earth would collapse. Without the control of earth, water will always flow to the lowest level. The internal links between the five elements maintain the balance between the five elements.

据《山海经》记载:"洪水滔天。鲧窃帝之息壤以堙洪水,不待帝命。帝令祝融杀鲧于羽郊。鲧复生禹,帝乃命禹卒布土以定九州。禹娶涂山氏女,不以私害公,自辛至甲四日,复往治水。"大禹吸取了父亲治水的教训,因势利导,治水成功,其实就是活用了五行生克之中的土克水的理论。

Legend in *The Classic of Mountains and Seas* has it that "During the reign of Emperor Yao, a rampant huge flood hit the villages in the Yellow River Valley. Gun stole some of the emperor's growing earth to withstand the devastating flood without the owner's permission. Because of this, Emperor Shun, who succeeded Yao, ordered Zhu Rong to kill Gun near the Yushan Mountain. Da Yu, as a posthumous child of Gun, was appointed by the emperor to follow in his father's footsteps. It was barely four days after he got married when he flung himself again into his career of fighting the flood." Da Yu learnt from his father's mistakes, taking the tide at the flood and dredging the river channels according to circumstances. Da Yu harnessed the flood with great success, which was a flexible application of the earth restricting water in the five elements theory.

五行之间的相互关系,正如《类经图翼》所载:"造化之机,不可无生,亦不可无制。无生则发育无由,无制则亢而为害。"相生和相克的关键在于相生和相克之间要达到平衡才能保证事物正常的生长和发展。为了保持两者的平衡,五行之间应既有相生,又有相克。

The relationship of the five elements, as is recorded in the *Leijing Tuyi*, "Neither generation nor restriction can be separated. Without inter-generation, there will be no growth and development; without inter-restriction, there will inevitably be abnormal hyperactivity which will consequently bring about harm." The key of inter-generation and inter-restriction lies in the relative balance between inter-generation and inter-restriction which ensures normal growth and development of things. To maintain balance between them, these elements are supposed to support one another (the generating cycle), and oppose one another (the controlling cycle).

(3) 相乘

乘,凌也,即乘虚侵袭、以强凌弱之意。五行相乘含有恃强欺弱的意思,类似于向弱的对手发起攻击。相乘是指五行中某一行本身太过,使原来克它的一行,不仅不能制约它,反而被它所克制,故又称反克。相乘是事物间的关系失却正常协调的一种表现。

③ Subjugation (Over-Restriction)

Invasion indicates encroaching on the weak counterpart. The demonstration of subjugation in relation to the five elements is "using one's strength to bully another one". Subjugation is similar to launching an attack when a counterpart is weak. It is an excessive restriction among the five elements. That is, one of the five elements becomes too excessive, thus the element that originally restricts it cannot restrict it anymore, but is restricted by it. Hence this is also known as subjugation (over-restriction), which is an abnormal manifestation in the normal coordinative relationship.

五行相乘的次序与相克的次序相同,即木乘土、土乘水、水乘火、火乘金、金乘木。引起五行之间相乘的原因,有"太过"和"不及"两个方面。"太过"所致的相乘,是指五行中某一行过于亢盛,对其所胜一行进行超过正常限度的克制,引起其所胜一行的虚弱,从而导致五行之间生克制化的异常。"不及"所致的相乘,是指五行中某一行过于虚弱,难以抵御其所不胜一行的正常限度的克制,使其本身更显虚弱。

Subjugation follows the order of restriction among the five elements: Wood subjugates earth, earth subjugates water, water subjugates fire, fire subjugates metal and metal subjugates wood. The possible reasons for subjugation are "being excessive" and "being deficient". Subjugation caused by "being excessive" means that one of the five elements is so hyperactive, strong and dominant that the restraint on its counterpart exceeds the normal limit, which causes the weakness of the counterpart, thus leading to the abnormal relation between the five elements. Subjugation caused by "being deficient" means that one of the five elements is so weak that the element that restricts is relatively hyperactive and will make excessive restriction on it.

以木克土为例,正常情况下,木克土,若木气过于亢盛,对土克制太过,则会导致土的不足,这种相乘现象,称为"木旺乘土"。仍以木克土为例,正常情况下,木能制约土,若土过于不足,即便木处于正常水平,土也仍然难以抵挡木的压制,因而导致木克土的力量相对增强,使土更显不足,这种相乘现象被称为"土虚木乘"。相乘与相克尽管在次序上相同,但两者是有区别的。相克是正常情况下五行之间依次制约的关系,相乘则是五行之间的异常制约关系。

For instance, wood normally restricts earth. However, if wood is in excess, it may over restrict earth and brings on insufficiency of earth. This situation is known as "wood subjugating earth". Take wood restricting earth as an example again, normally, wood restricts earth. If earth itself becomes weak, however, the strength of the restriction of earth by wood becomes relatively strengthened and it will further drain earth causing more deficiency. This is called "wood subjugates deficient earth". Although the order of subjugation is the same as that of restriction, there is a difference between them. Inter-restriction implies bringing under control or restraint among the five elements in a balanced normal environment. Subjugation is not a normal restriction but a harmful condition occurring under abnormal circumstances.

(4) 相侮

相侮,又称反侮,侮有欺凌、欺侮之意。从字面上讲,相侮就是依强欺弱。五行相侮,是指五行中某一行对其所不胜一行的反向克制,即反克。在病理条件下,一行不能按正常顺序克制另一行,反而被另一行克制。五行相侮的次序是:木侮金、金侮火、火侮水、水侮土、土侮木。五行相侮的次序与五行相克的次序相反。

① Counter-Restriction

Counter-restriction, also known as violation, is a kind of reversed restriction. Counter-restriction literally means that the strong one bullies the weak. Among the five elements it implies that one element counter-restricts another. It is a morbid condition in which one element fails to restrict the other in the regular order, but is restricted by the other in the reverse order. Counter-restriction follows such order among the five elements: Wood counter-restricts metal, metal counter-restricts fire, fire counter-restricts water, water counter-restricts earth, earth counter-restricts wood. Hence the order of counter-restriction is just the opposite to that of inter-restriction.

同相乘一样,引起五行之间相侮的原因也有"太过"和"不及"两个方面。"太过"所致的相侮,是指五行中的某一行过于强盛,使原来克制它的一行不仅不能克制它,反而受到它的反向克制。例如,正常情况下,金克木。但是当木盛金虚,木过于亢盛时,金不仅不能克木,反而会被木欺侮,出现"木反侮金"的逆向克制现象,这就叫作"木侮金"。"不及"所致的相侮,是指五行中某一行过于虚弱,不仅不能制约其所胜的一行,反而受到其所胜一行的反克。如正常情况下,木克土,但当木过度虚弱时,土会因木衰弱而反克之,这就叫作"土侮木"。

Just like subjugation, the possible reasons for counter-restriction lie in "being excessive" and "being deficient". Counter-restriction caused by "being excessive" means that one of the five elements is powerful and dominant, and as a result it is no longer controlled by the element that originally restricts it, but instead insults the element by restricting in the opposite direction. For example, under normal conditions, metal restricts wood. But when wood is in excess and metal is in deficiency, wood will counter-restrict metal instead of being restricted by metal, which is known as "wood counter-restricting metal". Counter-restriction caused by "being deficient" means that one of the five elements gets too weak, thus resulting in a relative strength of the element originally being restricted. Under normal conditions, for example, wood restricts earth. But when wood is of great weakness, earth will no longer be restricted by wood, but instead over-restricts the weakened wood in the opposite direction, that is what we call "earth counter-restricting wood".

（5）五行的母子关系

"母子相及"指五行中不正常的相生关系，包括"母病及子"和"子病及母"两个方面。"子病及母"的顺序和相克的顺序一样。

⑤ Mutual Interaction between Mother Organ and Child Organ

"Mother and child affecting each other" refers to abnormal intergeneration of the five elements. The interaction between mother organ and child organ includes both "disorder of mother-organ affecting child-organ" and "disorder of child-organ affecting mother-organ." "Disorder of child-organ affecting mother-organ" is just the order of inter-restriction.

四、五行学说在中医中的应用

中医应用五行学说来说明人体生理、病理的发展变化及其与外部环境的相互关系等，从而进行辨证论治,达到预防和治疗疾病的目的。五行学说在中医中的应用,主要是以五行的特性来分析说明人体脏腑、经络等结构组织的五行属性,以五行的生克制化来阐释脏腑、经络之间和各种生理功能之间的相互关系。

4. Application of the Five Elements Theory in TCM

The five elements theory has been applied to TCM, serving mostly to illustrate physiological and pathological development and changes in the human body, and the relation of the body to the external environment, etc. Thus treatment determination based on syndrome differentiation has always been able to reach the ends of disease prevention and treatment. When applied to TCM, the theory of five elements is aimed principally at analyzing and interpreting structure and tissues in the human body such as *zang-fu* organs and meridian system according to the properties of the five elements, and elucidating the mutual interplay among the *zang-fu* organs and meridian system as well as other multiple physiological functions via the generation, restriction, subjugation and counter-restriction relationships of the five elements.

就身体功能而言,五行与身体的每个器官相对应。五行的相生可用来说明五脏之间的相互滋生关系,而五行的相克可用来说明五脏之间的相互制约关系。

In terms of body functions, the five elements correspond to each organ of the human body. Generation in the five elements is frequently serviceable in explaining the intergeneration and mutual promotion relationships among the five *zang*-organs (heart, liver, spleen, lungs and kidneys), while restriction in the five elements can be employed to elucidate the inter-restriction relationships among the five *zang*-organs.

五行学说将人体的内脏分别归类到相应的五行,以五行的特性来说明五脏的生理功能。譬如,木有生长、升发、条达舒畅的特性,肝喜条达舒畅,有疏通气血、调畅情志的功能,故而肝属木;火有温热、升腾的特性,心阳具有温煦之功,故而心属火;土具有生化、承载、受纳的特性,脾主运化水谷、化生精微,为气血生化之源,故而脾属土;金具有清洁、肃降、收敛的特性,肺气以肃降为顺,故而肺属金;水具有滋润、下行、闭藏的特性,肾有藏精、主水的功能,故而肾属水。

  Each of the internal organs in the human body, according to the theory of five elements, pertains to one of the corresponding five elements. The characteristics of the five elements serve as an analogy to explain the physiological functions of the five *zang*-organs. For example, wood has characteristics of growing, ascending and developing freely, the liver prefers to grow freely and has the properties of promoting the flow of *qi* and blood as well as regulating emotion. Thus the liver pertains to wood. Fire possesses characteristics of warming and rising. The heart pumps blood to warm the body. Thus the heart pertains to fire. Earth bears characteristics of generating, holding and receiving. The spleen is responsible for transforming and transporting nutrients to all parts of the body, serving as the source of *qi* and blood. Thus the spleen pertains to earth. Metal develops characteristics of purifying, descending and astringing. The lung is marked by purifying and descending, thus the lung pertains to metal. Water adopts moistening, downward moving and closing as its hallmark traits. The kidney is in charge of storing essence and governing water, thus the kidney pertains to water.

  五行学说还可以阐释五脏之间相互滋生、促进的关系。肝生心恰如木生火,肝藏血以济心;心生脾恰如火生土,心阳对脾的温煦作用助脾运化;脾生肺恰如土生金,脾气布精于肺;肺生肾恰如金生水,肺气通调水道以助肾水;肾生肝恰如水生木,肾藏精以滋养肝血。

  The five elements theory also plays a role in elucidating the mutual nourishment and promotion among the five *zang*-organs. The liver nourishes the heart, the same as wood generates fire. The liver stores blood to support the heart. The heart nourishes the spleen, the same as fire generates earth. The heart yang warms the spleen, buttressing the transportation and transformation of the spleen. The spleen nourishes the lung, the same as earth generates metal. The essence distributed by spleen *qi* flows upward into the lung. The lung nourishes the kidney, the same as metal generates water. The lung *qi* flows downward, dredging, regulating water passage and bolstering the kidney water. The kidney nourishes the liver, the same as water generates wood. The kidney stores essence to tonify the liver blood.

五行的生克乘侮关系不仅可以说明在生理条件下脏腑之间的相互关系,亦可阐释在病理情况下脏腑之间的相互影响。

The generation, restriction, subjugation and counter-restriction relationships of the five elements have been pursuing a two-fold role in explaining the relationships among the internal organs physiologically, and expounding the interplay of the internal organs pathologically.

中医认为疾病是五行相互作用的外在反映。内脏有疾则必显现于外。正如朱丹溪在《丹溪心法》中所载:"有诸内者,必形诸外。"人体内脏的功能活动及其相互关系的异常变化,都可以从面色、脉象、声音和口味等方面反映出来。另外,疾病的发生和发展,也与内脏生克关系的异常有关。当身体的某种器官和对应的五行失衡时,另一种器官和对应的五行也会受到影响。如果五行中的一行和另一行之间存在着"太过"或"不及"的关系,身体就会失衡,最终导致疾病发生。中医旨在通过采取整体治疗的方法来重新获得身体的平衡。中医不是治标,而是治本。

One of the key carrier of TCM theory is that diseases are reflections of the interaction of the five elements. The disease inside the body will definitely find its manifestation outside. In Zhu Danxi's *Danxi Xinfa*, it states that "The inside disease in the body is bound to have an outside manifestation." Abnormal changes in functional activities of the viscera and their relationships in the body can all be reflected through complexion, pulse, voice and taste, etc.

What's more, the onset and development of diseases are related to the abnormal generation and restriction relationships among the viscera. When one of the organs and its corresponding element are out of balance, the impact of such imbalance will ripple to the rest and its associated element. Any excess or deficiency between one element and the other among the five elements will lead to imbalances and disharmony in the body, which will eventually give rise to diseases. TCM aims at regaining the balance by adopting a holistic treatment. Instead of just eliminating symptoms, TCM addresses the root cause of the disease.

五行中每种元素都有与之相对应的口味，而每种口味又对与其相对应的器官产生重要的影响。口味与人体器官密切相关，因此它与人体的关系十分重要，这种关系会以不同的方式来影响人体。譬如，甜味属土，与脾胃相关联。当一个人情绪低落、疲劳或有压力时，吃些甜食会感觉舒适一些。中医绵延发展了几千年，它源于中国一系列传统的医疗实践，贯穿这些医疗实践的主线就是基于阴阳学说和五行学说的平衡机体各种功能的理论体系。

Each of these five elements corresponds to its unique flavor, which will exert a significant effect on its corresponding organ in the body. Flavors and internal organs in the body go hand in hand. Therefore, the relationship between them weighs a lot for it affects the body in quite different ways. The sweet taste, for example, corresponds to the earth element which has links with the spleen and stomach. When one is feeling down, tired or stressed, his craving for sweet food will bring him comfort. TCM, whose history stretches back thousands of years, is a series of traditional medical practices which originated in China. The main thread running through these practices is the theoretical system that balances the various functions of the body based on the theory of yin-yang and the five elements.

第六章　气血津液

气、血、津液是构成和维持人体生命活动的基本物质。气,是人体内无形的、运行不息的极细微物质;血,是循行于脉中的红色液态物质;津液,是人体内的正常水液的总称。气、血、津液是脏腑、经络等器官组织生理活动的物质基础。

Chapter 6　*Qi*, Blood and Body Fluid

Qi, blood and body fluid are the basic substances which constitute and maintain life activities of human body. *Qi* is a kind of invisible, extremely tiny substance which moves unceasingly in the body; blood is the red liquid substance circulating in the blood vessel; body fluid is an umbrella term for the normal liquid inside the human body. *Qi*, blood and body fluid are the material basis for the physiological activities of *zang-fu* organs together with meridians and collaterals.

一、气

1. 气的基本概念

在中国传统文化中,气是个哲学概念。任何词或短语都无法充分捕捉到它的含义。就像阴阳一样,气的概念是中国文化和中医思想的基础。中医离不开中国传统文化,理解气要从理解中国传统文化开始。

1. Qi

(1) Fundamental Concept of Qi

Qi, in traditional Chinese culture, is originally a philosophical concept. No words or phrases can adequately capture its meaning. The notion of qi is as fundamental to Chinese culture and TCM thought as yin and yang. Approaching TCM is inseparable from getting closer to traditional Chinese culture, and our understanding of qi starts from the understanding of traditional Chinese culture.

对中国人而言,世间万物皆由气组成,并由气来定义。气是构成自然界最基本的物质。如《周易》所载:"天地氤氲,万物化醇。"宇宙间万物皆始于气的运动变化。它具有很强的活力和不断运动这两个特性。中医秉承了中国古代的传统文化和哲学思想,所以将人体内无形的而又真实存在的物质统称为气。

For the Chinese, everything in the universe is composed of and defined by qi. Qi serves as the most basic substance constituting the natural world. As recorded in Books of Changes, "When the chaotic yang qi from the heaven and yin qi from the earth roll into one, everything comes to being with pure nature." Everything in the universe begins with the constant motion and change of qi, which develops two features of strong vitality and constant movement. In TCM, the invisible but real substance in the human body is collectively called qi, which reflects the truth that TCM clings to traditional Chinese culture and philosophical thought firmly.

在中医里,气是个抽象的概念,中医典籍《黄帝内经》有云:"人以天地之气生,四时之法成。"人禀天地之气而生,天地合气,命之曰人。《黄帝内经·灵枢》曾载:"此四时之序,气之所处,病之所舍,藏之所宜。"气是维持生命活动的物质基础。气的运动变化伴随着能量的转换,被称之为气化,这是生命的基本特征。气化是血液生成的动力，正所谓"气为血之帅，血为气之母"，故而中医有"气行则血行"和"气滞则血瘀"的说法。

  Qi in TCM is an abstract concept. TCM classic *Inner Canon of the Yellow Emperor* states that "Man comes to life through the *qi* of heaven and earth. He matures in accordance with the laws of the seasons." The existence of human beings depends on the interaction between the celestial *qi* and terrestrial *qi*. As stated in *Spiritual Pivot* that "The needling methods are employed according to the order of the four seasons, the condition of *qi*, the location of diseases and the states of the *zang-fu* organs." *Qi* is the material base for life activities. The changes in its motion, accompanied by the energy transformation, is called *qihua* which is the basic feature of life. *Qihua* serves as the driving force for blood generation. The relationship between *qi* and blood is usually generalized as that "*qi* is the commander of blood and blood is the mother of *qi*". This is why there are sayings in TCM about the links between *qi* and blood, "normal flow of *qi* ensuring normal circulation of blood" and "stagnation of *qi* leading to stasis of blood".

  对于中国人来说，人的生命完全有赖于气。中医认为气乃人体之根，就如一棵树一般，一旦根部受损，茎叶势必无存。气并非原初的、一成不变的物质，也不仅仅是充满生命力的能量。气是贯穿生命万物的主线。宇宙因气的存在而运动不息。气是人存在和成长的基本特征，正如《黄帝内经·素问》所载："人有五脏化五气，以生喜怒悲忧恐。"气是生命的根源。故清初名医喻昌所撰写的《医门法律》有载："气聚则形成，气散则形亡。"

  For the Chinese, man's life relies entirely upon *qi*. *Qi* in TCM is the root of the human body. Just like a tree, once the root is damaged, the stem and leaves will naturally turn withered. *Qi* is not some primordial, immutable material, nor is it merely vigorous energy. It is the thread connecting everything. The universe moves ceaselessly due to its existence. *Qi* is the essential feature of being and becoming. As stated in *Plain Questions*, "In the human body the five *zang*-organs generate five kinds of visceral *qi* which give rise to the five emotions (joy, anger, contemplation, anxiety and fear)." *Qi* is the root of life. Therefore, Yu Chang, a renowned doctor in the early Qing Dynasty, said in his *Medical Laws* that "When *qi* gathers, the body will take shape; when *qi* disperses, the body will perish."

2. 气的来源

人体的气由三部分组成,即元气(秉承父母的先天之精气)、谷气(饮食中水谷精微所化生的水谷之气)和空气(肺部从自然界吸入的清气)。

(2) Origins of *Qi*

Qi in the body stems from three sources. The first of these is *yuanqi*, which is transmitted by parents to their children at conception. A second one is *guqi*, which is derived from the nutrients of water and food in diet. The third is *kongqi*, which is extracted by the lungs from the air we breathe.

气有先天之气和后天之气之分。出生前秉承父母的先天之精气,贮藏于肾,由肾精转化,称为"先天之气";出生后脾胃运化的水谷精微和肺部从自然界吸入的清气又被合称为"后天之气"。这三者通过肾、脾胃和肺等脏器生理功能的综合作用而生成,其中脾胃是关键。

Qi in the human body is interpreted as two aspects, allowing innate *qi* as well as acquired *qi*. The former is inherited from birth, stored in the kidney and transformed from the kidney essence, and the latter is acquired after birth, deriving from both food nutrients transformed by spleen-stomach and fresh air inhaled by the lung. The production of *qi* depends on the joint efforts of physiological functions of these viscera organs, such as the kidney, spleen, stomach and lung, among which the spleen and stomach are the key.

东汉王充在其所撰《论衡·气寿》中写道:"人之禀气,或充实而坚强,或虚劣而软弱。充实坚强,其年寿;虚劣软弱,失弃其身。天地生物,物有不遂;父母生子,子有不就。物有为实,枯死为堕;人有为儿,夭命而伤。使实不枯,亦至满岁;使儿不伤,亦至百年。然为实、儿而死枯者,禀气薄,则虽形体完,其虚劣气少,不能充也。儿生,号啼之声鸿朗高畅者寿,嘶喝湿下者夭。何则? 禀寿夭之命,以气多少为主性也。妇人疏字者子活,数乳者子死。何则? 疏而气渥,子坚强;数而气薄,子软弱也。"王充关于先天之气与寿命关系的论述,发人深省。

During the Eastern Han Dynasty, in Wang Chong's *On balance*, he wrote that "When a baby is endowed with innate *qi* inherited from parents, he or she will be strong if there is adequate *qi*. Otherwise, the baby will be born weak. A man with adequate *qi* lives a long life while a man with scanty *qi* is just the other way around. Heaven and earth produce all things, but some fail to thrive. Parents give birth to children, but some can't grow up. Some fruits wither and fall down; some children die at birth. Suppose the fruits were still fresh, they would grow till the end. Suppose the baby was still alive, he would live to be a hundred. In view of the scanty *qi*, actually the reverse is true. Even if their bodies are complete, the innate *qi* still can't suffuse in the body if one is born weak with insufficient *qi* inside the body. A baby can live long if he cries loudly, sonorously and unimpededly when he is born and short if he cries exhaustedly, lowly and feebly. Why is this? One's life span depends on the amount of innate *qi*. Children with sub-fertile mothers are inclined to survive easily, while those with productive mothers tend to die young. Why? A child can receive more sufficient innate *qi* if he has fewer brothers and sisters, and the opposite goes the other way around." Wang Chong's remarks on the relationship between innate *qi* and life span are thought-provoking.

3. 气的运动

气和运动不可分割。气具有很强的活力,不停地在人体中运动以维持人体的正常生理功能。气的不断运动叫作"气机"。气的运动方式从理论上来讲可归纳为升、降、出、入四种基本类型。升,是指气自下而上的运动;降,是指气自上而下的运动;出,是指气由内向外的运动;入,是指气由外向内的运动。气的升降运动是普遍存在、运行不息的。中医常以气的运动变化来阐释人体的生命活动。

(3) Movements of *Qi*

Qi, which is in separable from movement, is in constant motion with full vitality so as to maintain the body's normal physiological functions. Such an unceasing trend of motion is known as *qiji*. The various forms of its movement may be theoretically summarized under four main categories—ascending, descending, exiting and entering. Ascending, for example, is a kind of motion of *qi* from lower to upper, while descending is just the opposite direction. Exiting means that *qi* moves from interior to exterior, while entering of *qi* moves just the other way around. The motion of *qi* exists universally and ceaselessly. It's frequently the case that TCM elucidates life activities of the human body via the movement of *qi*.

津液的生成、输布及排泄依赖气的升、降、出、入运动。人体的脏腑、经络等器官组织,都是气的升降出入场所。经脉是气在身体各部位流动的隐形通道。没有气的升降就没有转化、吸收和贮藏,没有气的出入就没有生长和发展。气的升降出入运动,是人体生命活动的根本,一旦停止,也就意味着生命的终结。

The generation, distribution and discharge of body fluid depend on the ascending, descending, exiting and entering of *qi*. The organs and tissues in the body, such as *zang-fu* organs, meridians and collaterals are all places where *qi* moves in and out. Passages are invisible pathways through which *qi* circulates in all parts of the body. Without ascending and descending of *qi*, there will be no transformation, absorption, and storing. Without exiting and entering of *qi*, there will be no growth and development. What at the bottom of human life activities is the movement of *qi*. Once it stops, it means an end of life.

就整个人体的生理活动而言,气的升降出入必须协调平衡,如此方能维持正常的生理活动。中医把气的升降出入的协调平衡状态称作"气机调畅";把气的升降出入的阻塞失调状态称作"气机失调"。

In terms of the physiological activity of the whole body, normal physiological activities of the body demand coordination and balance between ascending, descending, exiting and entering of *qi*. In TCM, a coordinated and balanced state of *qi* movement is known as "harmony of *qi* activity". Conversely, an obstruction and disharmony of *qi* movement is known as "disorder of *qi* activity".

4. 气的分类

中医认为气有诸多种类。然而这诸多类别的气,归根结底属于同一种气,只不过表现形式不同而已。根据它们的组成、分布和功能,气可以分为四类,即元气、宗气、营气和卫气。

(4) Classification of *Qi*

TCM deems that there are various kinds of *qi*. All these various kinds of *qi*, however, will be ultimately boiled down to one same kind of *qi*, merely manifesting in different forms. This only one *qi* assumes four different categories, namely primordial *qi*, pectoral *qi*, nutrient *qi* and defensive *qi* according to their composition, distribution and functions.

元气,又名"原气",是人体最根本、最重要的气。元气主要由肾中精气化生而来。它以先天精气为基础,辅以后天水谷精气的补给。因此,元气的盛衰并不完全取决于先天禀赋,也与后天脾胃运化水谷精微的功能密切相关。元气发于肾,通过三焦循行全身,内则经历五脏六腑,外则达肌肤腠理,无所不至。

Primordial *qi*, also known as "original *qi*", is the most fundamental and important *qi* of the human body. Primordial *qi* comes mainly from the innate essence stored in the kidney. It has largely been based on congenital endowments, but it also requires the replenishment of food nutrients essence transformed by spleen-stomach. Therefore, the wax and wane of primordial *qi* depends not only entirely on nature, but also on nurture. Primordial *qi* stems from the kidney essence, and flows throughout the body via *sanjiao* (triple energizer), going inward to the viscera and outward to the muscle as well as skin with an all-pervasive nature.

宗气指积于胸中的后天之气。宗气在胸中积聚之处,被称作"气海"。宗气是由肺部从自然界吸入的清气和脾胃从饮食中运化的水谷精气结合而成。后者为宗气的主要组成部分。肺的呼吸功能、脾胃的水谷精微运化功能与宗气的盛衰密切相关。

The acquired pectoral *qi* gathers in the chest, where it forms a "sea of *qi*". Pectoral *qi*, which is mainly derived from both fresh air inhaled by the lung and food essence transformed by spleen-stomach, takes the latter part as its mainstay. Respiratory function of the lung, together with the transportation and transforming functions of the spleen and stomach, is closely linked with the vitality of the pectoral *qi*.

《黄帝内经》曾载这种宗气"走息道以司呼吸,贯心脉以行气血"。宗气积聚于胸中,灌注于心肺,其主要功能是帮助调节呼吸的强弱、心搏的节律。呼吸、声音、心跳、气血的运行,皆与宗气的盛衰相关。

According to *Inner Canon of the Yellow Emperor*, pectoral *qi* "goes through the respiratory tract to move respiration, and connects the heart and vessels to propel the flow of *qi*". The main function of pectoral *qi*, which gathers in the chest and connects the heart together with the lungs, aims to assist the regulation of the respiration intensity (forceful or weak) and rhythm of the heartbeat. The respiration, voice, heartbeat, and the movement of *qi* and blood, are all related to the wax and wane of pectoral *qi*.

营气,是指循行于脉中具有营养作用的气,又称"荣气"。由于营气与血可分而不可离,故常以"营血"相称。营气运行于血脉之中,帮助化生水谷精微,是为人体提供营养的要素。

Nutritive *qi*, also known as "*rongqi*", circulates within the vessels with a nutritive function. Since nutritive *qi* and blood seem to blend into one, they are often called "nutritive blood" for they allow an explicit separation possible but an implicit total break-up of both impossible. Nutritive *qi*, which moves in the blood vessels and supports the transportation together with transformation of food essence, is an essential factor for body nourishment.

卫气护卫肌表,防御外邪入侵。营气和卫气都源自水谷精微,但是"营在脉中""卫在脉外"。营气属阴,卫气属阳,故又有"营阴""卫阳"之称。

Defensive *qi* serves as a guardian of the surface layer structure of human body, warding off the invasion of exogenous pathogenic factors. Although nutritive *qi* and defensive *qi* both stem from the food essence, they differ a lot in that the nutritive *qi* flows inside the vessel while the defensive *qi* flows outside the vessel. Nutritive *qi* pertains to yin, while defensive *qi* belongs to yang. This explains why they get the labels of "nutritive yin" and "defensive yang" respectively.

5. 气的功能

作为维持人体生命活动的最基本物质,气对人体具有十分重要的功能。

(5) Functions of *Qi*

As the most basic substance in sustaining body activities, *qi* performs significant functions.

气是不断运动着的具有很强活力的精微物质,它对于人体的生长发育及脏腑、经络等组织器官的生理活动,血的生成和运行,津液的生成、输布和排泄等,均起着推动和激发其运行的作用。人体之气充盈,生理活动就完好正常。人体之气虚衰,就会出现诸如无精打采等症状。

As a refined constant moving substance with strong vitality, *qi* plays a propelling and invigorating role in sustaining body activities, ranging from the growth, development and reproduction of the body, physiological activities of tissues and organs such as viscera and meridians, the production and circulation of blood to the generation, excretion and distribution of body fluid, etc. When *qi* is abundant, physiological activities of the body will be sound and normal. Conversely, when *qi* is deficient, symptoms such as lethargy and exhaustion will arise.

气是人体产生热量的物质基础。人的体温,脏腑、经络的生理活动皆依赖气的温煦作用来维持。据《难经》记载:"气主煦之。"人体生理功能的正常发挥,有赖于气的温煦作用;血和津液等液态物质的正常运行,也要依靠气的温煦作用。所以有"血得温而行,得寒而凝"之说。

Qi serves as the material basis for heat generation of the body. The constant body temperature, together with physiological activities of *zang-fu* organs, meridians and collaterals all depend on the warming function of *qi*. As stated in *Classic of Medical Difficulties*, "*Qi* performs a warming function." Only through the warming function of *qi*, can physiological activities of human body work normally. The warming function of *qi* is an essential prerequisite for the normal circulation of blood, body fluid, etc. Therefore, as the saying goes, "Blood flows when it gets warm, but coagulates when it gets cold."

气的防御作用,主要体现在护卫全身的肌表和防御外邪的入侵,是机体抗病能力的体现。《黄帝内经·素问》曰:"正气存内,邪不可干。""邪之所凑,其气必虚。"人体之气旺盛,则不易受邪气侵害。如果气的防御作用减弱,外邪就容易侵入机体,从而引发疾病。

The defending function of *qi*, which is the embodiment of the body's disease resistance, is mainly reflected in guarding the surface layer structure of human body, and fighting against the invasion of the exogenous pathogenic factors. As stated in *Plain Questions*, "Invasion of pathogenic evil *qi* will get nowhere as long as sufficient healthy vital *qi* exists inside the body." "The accumulation of evil *qi* leads to the deficiency of *qi*." With sufficient *qi* exists inside the body, the exogenous pathogenic factors have no way to invade. If *qi* gets weak, however, the exogenous pathogenic factors tend to penetrate the body easily. Hence illness will naturally arise.

气的固摄作用,主要指气对体内精、血、汗、津液等液态物质具有防止其无故流失的作用。

The consolidating function of *qi* mainly refers to the effect of preventing liquid substances such as sperm, blood, sweat, body fluid from extravasation and losing unduly.

气的气化作用,是指由于气的运动产生的精、气、血、津液的新陈代谢及其相互转化。譬如,人体将水谷精微化生成气、血、津液,津液经过代谢,转化成汗液和尿液,食物被消化和吸收后,其残渣转化成糟粕等,这些都是气化作用的具体体现。因此,气化作用的过程,就是物质代谢与能量转化的过程。

The function of *qihua* (*qi* transforming) is a matter of the metabolism and mutual transformation of essence, *qi*, blood and body fluid due to the movement of *qi*. The production of *qi*, blood and body fluid, for example, depends on the transformation of food essence. Body fluid is converted into sweat and urine by means of metabolism. After digestion and absorption, the residues of food are turned into feces, etc. All these processes are concrete manifestations of the transforming activity of *qi*. Thus the process of *qihua* is a process of material metabolism and energy conversion.

二、血

1. 血的基本概念

血,是循行于脉管之中的富有营养的红色液态物质,是构成和维持人体生命活动的基本物质之一。脉是血液循行的管道,被称为"血之府"。脉道的完好无损与畅通无阻是保证血液正常循行的重要因素。

2. Blood

(1) Fundamental Concept of Blood

Blood is a nutritious red liquid substance circulating within the blood vessels and one of the basic substances constituting and maintaining human life activities. The vessel, known as "the house of blood", is the channel through which blood flows. The intact and smooth vessels are key factors in ensuring the normal blood circulation.

2. 血的生成

血主要由营气和津液组成。营气和津液源自经脾胃运化而生成的水谷精微。在这个过程中,脾胃的生理功能尤为重要。如果脾胃虚弱,不能运化水谷精微,或化源不足,则会导致血虚。临床上治疗血虚,首先要调理脾胃,故而脾胃是气血生化之源。肾藏精,倘若精气丰沛,肾中所藏之精可能会转化为血,而当血液充盈之时,血亦有可能转化为精,故有"精血同源"之说。

(2) Generation of Blood

Blood is mainly composed of the nutritive *qi* and body fluid which come from the food essence via the transportation and transformation of spleen-stomach. During this process, the physiological function of the spleen-stomach plays a vital role. A weak spleen-stomach fails to transport and transform food essence, or gives rise to a poor transformation, hence blood deficiency occurs. Clinical treatment of blood deficiency, more often than not, starts from regulating the spleen and stomach. Therefore, it is said that spleen and stomach are the source of *qi* and blood. Kidney stores essence. When the essence stored in the kidney is sufficient, it may transform into blood. When blood is abundant, it may in turn transform into essence. Hence there is a saying that "The essence and blood share the same origin."

3. 血的循环

血液在脉管中以"阴阳相贯,如环无端"的方式运行不息、环周不休。血的运行受多种因素的影响,也是多个脏腑功能共同作用的结果。

(3) Circulation of Blood

Blood circulates ceaselessly in the vessels, connecting yin and yang end by end and spreading over the whole body like "a ring without an end". Being influenced by numerous factors, blood circulation is a result of the joint efforts of *zang-fu* functions.

血属阴而主静,血的运行主要依赖气的推动。气的固摄作用使血行脉中而不致逸出脉外。气的推动与固摄作用、温煦与防御作用之间的平衡协调是血液正常运行的基本保障。

The blood belongs to yin with the feature of quiescence. Blood circulation mainly depends on the propelling power of qi. Relying on the controlling function of qi, blood circulation will confine itself within the vessels instead of overflowing the vessels. The balance and coordination between these functions of qi—the propelling and controlling functions, together with the warming and defending functions, are the basic guarantee which ensures a smooth blood circulation.

血液的循行,与脏腑器官诸如心、肺、肝、脾等的功能密切相关。心主血脉,充足的心气在血液循环中起主导作用,推动血液在脉中循行。正如《黄帝内经·素问·经脉别论》所载,"肺朝百脉",这是对气、血、心肺关系的高度概括。肺吐故纳新,调节人体气机,完成人体内外的气体交换。肝主疏泄,能调畅情志,还能贮藏血液,调节血量。血液的循环离不开心气的推动、肺气的宣发以及肝气的疏泄。脾主统血,脾气健旺则气血旺盛。脾气的统摄功能及肝气的藏血功能都是血液循行的保障。

The circulation of the blood is closely related to the function of *zang-fu* organs such as the heart, lung, liver and spleen, etc. The heart governs the blood and vessels. Sufficient heart *qi*, which propels the blood to circulate in the vessels, plays a leading role in blood circulation. A quote from *Plain Questions* highly sums up the relationship between *qi*, blood, heart and lung, "All vessels converge in lung." By exhaling the stale and inhaling the fresh, the lung regulates *qi* function and accomplishes the exchange of *qi* inside and outside the human body. Liver performs multiple roles, ranging from governing dispersion and catharsis, regulating emotions, storing blood to regulating blood volume. Blood circulation cannot be divorced from the propelling function of the heart-*qi*, the dispersing function of the lung-*qi* and the distributing function of the liver-*qi*. The spleen governs blood. Healthy and vigorous spleen *qi* yields to exuberant *qi* and blood. The governing function of the spleen-*qi* and the storing function of the liver-*qi* are all guarantees for blood circulation.

4. 血的功能

血主要有营养和滋润全身的功能。《黄帝内经·素问·五脏生成》曰:"肝受血而能视,足受血而能步,掌受血而能握,指受血而能摄。"血在脉中循行,为脏腑提供营养,确保脏腑发挥生理功能,保证人体生命活动的正常进行。

(4) Functions of Blood

Blood mainly has a pivotal role to play in nourishing and moistening the whole body. As stated in *Plain Questions*: *Discussion on Various Relationships Concerning the Five Zang-Organs*, "Blood will be the biggest nourishment for the liver which enables the eyes to see, for the feet to walk, for the palm to grasp, and for the fingers to take." Circulating in the vessels, blood plays a three-fold role—providing nutrition for the viscera, guaranteeing physiological functions of viscera, and ensuring normal life activities of human body.

三、津液

1. 津液的基本概念

津液是人体一切正常水液的总称,涵盖各脏腑组织器官的正常体液及正常分泌物,如唾液、胃液、肠液及尿、汗、涕、泪等。同气血一样,津液也是构成和维持人体生命活动的基本物质之一。

3. Body Fluid

(1) Fundamental Concept of Body Fluid

Body fluid is a collective name for all normal liquids in human body, covering normal internal body fluids of *zang-fu* organs, tissues and normal excretions, such as saliva, gastric juice, intestinal juice together with urine, sweat, nasal discharge and tears, etc. Just like *qi* and blood, body fluid is one of the basic substances constituting and maintaining life activities.

津和液,既有区别又有联系。二者同属水液,均来源于饮食水谷,无一例外有赖脾胃的运化功能。但二者在性状、分布部位和功能方面的区别又无可否认。《黄帝内经·灵枢·决气》曰:"何谓津?……腠理发泄,汗出溱溱,是谓津。何谓液?……谷入气满,淖泽注入骨,骨属屈伸,泄泽补益脑髓,皮肤润泽,是谓液。"通常来说,津质地清稀,一个显著特点是其流动性大;而液质地浓稠,流而不行。津液各走其道,津分布于体表皮肤、肌肉和孔窍;而液则灌注于脑髓、骨节、脏腑等。津能渗入血脉,起滋润作用;而液则起濡养作用。由于二者同属水液,可以相互转化,故津和液时常并称。

Jin (thin fluid) and *ye* (thick fluid) are two different but related concepts. They share one quality—they both belong to body fluid. Relying upon transportation and transformation functions of spleen-stomach without exception, they both derive from food and water. Yet big differences in properties, distributions and functions between them are undeniable. A quote from *Spiritual Pivot*: *Differentiation of Qi* highly sums up the distinction between *jin* (thin fluid) and *ye* (thick fluid), "What is *jin* (thin fluid)?....When *couli* (muscular interstices) opens, the body is drenched with sweat. This is the so-called *jin* (thin fluid). What is *ye* (thick fluid)?.... When food and water are taken into the stomach, the essence-qi arising from this spreads over the whole body and plays multiple roles. It not only infuses into the bones, enabling the bones to flex and extend smoothly, but infuses into the body to tonify the brains and moisten the skin. This is known as *ye* (thick fluid)." Generally speaking, *jin* (thin fluid) is thin and lucid. One of the most striking characteristics of *jin* (thin fluid) involves moving with more fluidity. While *ye* (thick fluid) is thick and turbid. It flows with less fluidity but not spreads. *jin* (thin fluid) and *ye* (thick fluid) go their ways separately. *Jin* (thin fluid) is distributed over the body's surface layer structure, skin, muscles and orifices. While *ye* (thick fluid) perfuses into and tonifies brain and marrow, joints and viscera, etc. *Jin* (thin fluid) spreads over and seeps into the blood vessels to moisten the body. While *ye* (thick fluid) plays a part in nourishing the body. *Jin* (thin fluid) and *ye* (thick fluid), more often than not, are equivalents of each other for they both pertain to body fluid and tend to transform into each other under certain conditions.

2. 津液的代谢

津液的生成、输布和排泄涉及多个脏腑器官的生理功能,津液的代谢过程是多个脏腑器官相互协调配合的结果。正如《黄帝内经·素问·经脉别论》所载:"饮入于胃,游溢精气,上输于脾;脾气散精,上归于肺,通调水道,下输膀胱。水精四布,五经并行。"这段话通常被认为是对人体津液代谢过程的高度概括。

(2) Metabolism of Body Fluid

The formation, distribution and excretion of body fluid come down to the physiological functions of multiple *zang-fu* organs. The process of body fluid metabolism is exactly the result of coordination and cooperation of multiple viscera. As stated in *Plain Questions: Special Discussion on Channels and Vessels*, "When body fluid is formed in the stomach, the essence-*qi* spreads, overflows and ascends into the spleen. The spleen plays a role in dispersing the essence, and the body fluid ascends into the lung via the lung's dispersing. The lung regulates water passage through its descending function, and the body fluid descends into the bladder. In this way, water-essence spreads over the body and the five meridians move together." This passage is usually considered to be epitome and highlight of the process of body fluid metabolism.

津液的生成与脾、胃、小肠、大肠等脏腑器官的生理活动密切相关。津液源于饮食水谷,通过脾、胃、小肠和大肠的消化吸收生成。胃为水谷之海,胃气吸收水谷之精微。脾主运化,将肠胃所吸收的水谷精微上输至心肺,继而输布全身。

The formation of body fluid goes hand in hand with the physiological activities of *zang-fu* organs such as the spleen, stomach, small intestine and large intestine, etc. The body fluid, which stems from food and water in diet, is formed through digesting and absorbing food essence via spleen, stomach, small intestine and large intestine. Stomach is known as the sea of the food essence, which is received and absorbed by the stomach-*qi*. Spleen, a governor for transportation and transformation, ascends the food essence to the heart and lung, and then spreads them over the whole body.

津液的输布和排泄主要是通过脾、肺、肾和三焦等脏腑器官生理功能的协调配合来实现。脾主运化,正如《黄帝内经·素问·至真要大论》所载:"诸湿肿满,皆属于脾。"脾将津液上输至肺,通过肺的宣发肃降,将津液布散全身。肺主行水,通调水道,故而肺又被称为"水之上源"。肾为水脏,推动和调控人体津液的输布和排泄。津液在体内的输布和排泄有赖于多个脏腑器官生理功能的相互配合、相互协调。

The distribution and excretion of body fluid is mainly realized by the coordination of the physiological functions of the *zang-fu* organs such as spleen, lung, kidney and triple energizer, etc. Spleen governs transportation and transformation. As stated in *Plain Questions*, "The symptoms such as dampness and swelling, by and large, affiliate themselves with the abnormal function of the spleen." Spleen conveys the body fluid up to the lung, and then spreads the body fluid over the whole body via the lung's dispersing and descending functions. The lung is also known as "the upper source of water" for it governs water circulation and regulates water passage. The kidney, also known as the water organ, propels and regulates the distribution and excretion of body fluid. The distribution and excretion of body fluid rely upon the interaction and coordination of the physiological functions of multiple *zang-fu* organs.

津液的输布和排泄涉及肾、肺、脾等多个脏腑器官。其中,肾在维持人体津液代谢平衡中起着至关重要的作用。

The distribution and excretion of body fluid involve multiple *zang-fu* organs, such as kidney, lung, spleen, etc. Among them, kidney plays a critical role in maintaining metabolic balance of body fluid.

总而言之,津液的生成、输布和排泄是通过诸多脏腑器官相互协调、相互配合来实现的,尤以脾、肺、肾之间的协调最重要。

To sum up, the formation, distribution and excretion of body fluid are realized by the coordination and cooperation of multiple organs, especially the coordination of the spleen, lungs, and kidneys.

3. 津液的功能

津液内含营养物质,有滋润濡养人体脏腑组织器官和化生血液的功能。这些功能相辅相成、不可分割。

津液渗入脉中为血液,溢出脉外为津液。津液和血液都是由水谷精微化生而成,故有"津血同源"之说。

(3) Functions of Body Fluid

Body fluid claims to contain nutritious substances, performing multiple complementary and inseparable functions of moistening, nourishing the *zang-fu* organs and tissues, and generating blood. Body fluid turns into blood when infiltrating into the vessels, and transforms into body fluid when overflowing out of the vessels. Both body fluid and blood stem from food essence, hence there is the saying "body fluid and blood are of the same origin".

津液的代谢还可以调节身体内外环境的平衡。当天气炎热时,津液化为汗液向外排泄以散热;当天气寒冷时,津液闭而不泄以维持体温。

The metabolism of body fluid can also regulate the balance of the internal and external environments of the body. When the weather is hot, body fluid turns into sweat excreting outwards to dissipate heat. While when the weather is cold, body fluid shuts but not release so as to maintain body temperature.

四、气、血、津液之间的关系

气、血、津液之间存在着相互渗透、相互依存、相互作用的密切关系。

4. Relationships between *Qi*, Blood and Body Fluid

Qi, blood and body fluid have a close relationship of interpenetration, interdependence and interaction.

气与血关系密切,中医将两者之间的关系概括为:"气为血之帅,血为气之母。"气对血有统率作用,是血液生成和循行的动力,血能养气,亦能载气。血是气的载体和化生基础。《难经·二十二难》曰:"气主煦之,血主濡之。"气属阳,津液属阴。气和津液之间的关系类似于气和血的关系。

There is a close affinity between *qi* and blood. In TCM, the relationship between the two is summarized as "*Qi* is the commander of blood, and blood is the mother of *qi*." As the driving force of blood generation and circulation, *qi* has a commanding effect on blood. Blood, which is the basis and carrier of *qi* generation, can nourish *qi*, and it can also carry *qi*. According to *Classic of Medical Difficulties*, "*Qi* governs warming, and blood governs nourishing." *Qi* belongs to yang, while body fluid pertains to yin. The relationship between *qi* and body fluid is similar to *qi* and blood.

血和津液都由水谷精微化生而来,故有"津血同源"之说,血和津液都具有滋润濡养的作用,它们之间存在着相互依存、相互转化的关系。

Both blood and body fluid derive from food essence. Hence it is said that "body fluid and blood are of the same origin". Both of them have important roles to play in moistening and nourishing, and there is a relationship of mutual dependence and mutual transformation between them.

《吕氏春秋·尽数》中有段话阐释了气、血、津液和运动养生之间的关系:"流水不腐,户枢不蝼,动也。形气亦然。形不动则精不流,精不流则气郁。郁处头则为肿为风,处耳则为挶为聋,处目则为蔑为盲,处鼻则为鼽为窒,处腹则为张为疛,处足则为痿为蹷。"

An excerpt from *Spring and Autumn Annals of Lv Buwei* elucidates the relationship between *qi*, blood, body fluid, exercise and health cultivation: "A running stream never goes stale and a rotating door-hinge never erodes easily. This is why human body must have physical exercises. The same is true of the relationship between physical body and *qi*. A lack of exercise will give rise to unsmooth circulation of essence, which in its turn leads to a stagnation of *qi*. If the accumulated *qi* moves to the head, there will be a swelling in the head and face; if it moves to ears, there will be earache or deafness; if it moves to eyes, there will be sore eyes or blindness; if it moves to the nose, there will be rhinalgia or nasal congestion; if it moves to the abdomen, there will be abdominal distension or pain; and if it moves to feet, there will be foot ache or shriveled feet."

第七章　藏象学说

中医对脏腑器官生理、病理的认识,传统上称为"藏象学说"。"藏象"这个术语首先出现在《黄帝内经·素问·六节藏象论》:"脏象何如?"藏,中医是指藏于体内的脏腑器官;象,是指表现于外的生理、病理现象。藏是象的内在本质,象是藏的外在反映,两者合起来就叫作"藏象"。正如明代张景岳的《类经》所载:"象,形象也。脏居于内,形见于外,故曰脏象。"

Chapter 7　Theory of Visceral Manifestation

In TCM, the awareness of the *zang-fu* organs' physiological and pathological phenomenon is traditionally called *zang xiang* theory (the theory of visceral manifestation). The term "*zang xiang*" (visceral manifestation) first appears in the *Chapter of Six Sections of Discussion on Zang Xiang* in *Plain Questions*: "How about *zang xiang* (viscera and their manifestations)?" *Zang* refers to the internal organs hidden inside the body, and *xiang* means the external manifestations of physiological and pathological phenomenon. *Zang* is the intrinsic nature of *xiang*, and *xiang* is the extrinsic reflection of *zang*. A combination of both is called "*zang xiang*". Just like *The Classified Classic* by Zhang Jingyue states that "*Xiang* (manifestation) refers to image. The viscera are stored inside the body and the image is manifested outwardly. Therefore, it is called visceral manifestation."

中医可以通过观察外在表象了解内脏的情况,比如可以通过一个人眼睛明亮与否、视物清晰与否来判断此人是否肝血充足;通过舌尖是否发红或糜烂来判断是否心火旺盛。这正如朱丹溪所说的那样:"欲知其内者,当以观乎外,诊于外者,斯以知其内,盖有诸内者形诸外。"这就是为什么外在的病变要调理内在脏腑。

TCM gets to know the condition of internal organs by observing the external manifestations. For instance, one can judge whether a person has sufficient liver blood by signs of bright eyes and clear vision; and one can judge whether a person has flaring of heart-fire by red tip of tongue or erosion of tongue. Just as Zhu Danxi states that "Inspection of the exterior manifestations will enable one to know the interior conditions; and diagnosis of the exterior will enable one to know the interior. This is because the interior can be manifested by the exterior." That is why the internal organs should be regulated for external diseases.

藏象学说是在长期临床实践的基础上逐渐形成和发展起来的。《黄帝内经·灵枢·经水》中的记载再现了当时基于人体器官观察的人体解剖的情景:"若夫八尺之士,皮肉在此,外可度量切循而得之,其死可解剖而视之。其脏之坚脆,腑之大小,谷之多少,脉之长短,血之清浊……皆有大数。"正是这些解剖学知识概括了人体的生理和病理学概念,奠定了藏象学说的形态基础。

Theory of *zang xiang* has been gradually formed and developed on the basis of long-term clinical practice. Records from *Spiritual Pivot* reproduced the scene of human anatomy based on observation of human organs at that time, "The eight-*chi* body-surface may be measured for the flesh is well within the reach of measurement. After death, the body can be dissected to observe the texture of the *zang*-organs (hard or crisp), the size of the *fu*-organs (big or small), the amount of food consumed (more or less), the length of the channels (long or short), the condition of the blood (clear or turbid), etc. All these can be roughly obtained via such hands-on dissection experience of the corpse." It is such knowledge of anatomy that generalizes the physiological and pathological concepts of human body, thus laying the morphological foundation of *zang xiang* theory.

心、肝、脾、肺、肾合称五脏,属于实体性器官。心主血脉,推动、调控心脏搏动而行血。中医认为,心脏居于五脏之首,起着主宰人体生命活动的作用。心脏的主要功能是心主血脉和心藏神。肝能贮藏血液,素有"血海"之称。肝主疏泄,调畅气机,舒畅情绪。脾主运化水谷,控制、统领血液运行。肺主宣发肃降,主持呼吸,通调水道,全身的气血通过经脉朝会于肺。《黄帝内经·素问·逆调论》记载:"肾者水脏,主津液。"肾藏精,主生长发育和生殖。

The heart, liver, spleen, lungs and kidneys, which fall into the category of substantive organs, are collectively called the five *zang*-organs. The heart, which governs blood vessels, propels and regulates heartbeat so as to facilitate blood circulation. In TCM, the heart has been given a high-priority rating among the five *zang*-organs for it plays a dominant role in life activities. The main physiological functions of the heart are that the heart governs blood vessels and stores spirit. The liver has long been known as the "blood sea" for it stores blood. Not only does it govern dispersion and distribution, regulate the *qi* activities, but it smoothes emotions. The spleen is multifunctional for it takes charge of transporting and transforming nutrients of water and food, controlling and governing blood circulation. The lung holds several posts simultaneously. It has a leading role in dominating dispersing, diffusion, purification and descent, commanding respiration and smoothing water passage. All vessels converge in the lung. *Qi* and blood of the whole body gather in the lungs through channels and vessels. As stated in the chapter *Discussion on Disharmony* in *Plain Questions*, "Being an organ of water, the kidney controls fluids." Storing essence, together with governing growth and reproduction are key features of the kidney.

五脏的共同生理特点是化生和贮藏精气。故而《黄帝内经·素问·五脏别论》有载:"所谓五脏者,藏精气而不泻也,故满而不能实。"无独有偶,唐代医学家王冰也有类似的表述:"精气为满,水谷为实。五脏但藏精气,故满而不实;六腑则不藏精气,但受水谷,故实而不能满也。"

The common physiological characteristics of the five *zang*-organs are to transform and store essence. Hence *Special Discussion on Five Zang-Organs* in *Plain Questions* states that "The so called five *zang*-organs store essence but not excrete it; that is the reason why they can be full but not solid." Coincidentally, Wang Bing, a distinguished physician in the Tang Dynasty, also made a similar statement, "Essence is characterized by fullness and food by solidity. The five *zang*-organs only store essence, hence they can just be full but not solid; the six *fu*-organs receive food but do not store essence, hence they can only be solid but not full."

中医认为,五脏和自然界四时阴阳相对应。正如《黄帝内经·素问·金匮真言论》所载:"五脏应四时。"关于四时,据《黄帝内经·素问·宝命全形论》记载:"人以天地之气生,四时之法成。""四时"即春、夏、秋、冬四个季节,每个季节各有特点,春温、夏热、秋凉、冬寒。不同的季节,对人体五脏的影响也不同。在《黄帝内经·素问·脏气法时论》里有肝主春、心主夏、脾主长夏、肺主秋、肾主冬的记载。五脏要顺应四时的自然规律,循天时之变,与外在环境取得协调一致,身体才能健康。

TCM believes that the five *zang*-organs correspond to the variations of the four seasons and yin-yang changes. As stated in *Plain Questions*, "The five *zang*-organs correspond to the four seasons." As regards the four seasons, *Plain Questions* gives relevant recording, "One comes to this world through the *qi* of heaven and earth, and he grows up in accordance with the law of the four seasons." Spring, summer, autumn and winter are four seasons in a year, which have their unique characteristics. Spring is warm, summer is hot, autumn is cool, and winter is cold. Different seasons exert different effects on the five *zang*-organs of the human body. As stated in *Plain Questions*, the liver corresponds to spring, the heart to summer, the spleen to the late summer, the lung to autumn and the kidney to winter. Only if the five *zang*-organs comply with natural laws of the four seasons, follow the changes of nature, and achieve harmony of the internal and external environment of the body will one be able to keep fit and stay healthy.

《黄帝内经·素问·六节脏象论》对此有着详细的记载:"心者,生之本,神之处也;其华在面,其充在血脉,为阳中之太阳,通于夏气。肺者,气之本,魄之处也;其华在毛,其充在皮,为阳中之太阴,通于秋气。肾者，主蛰，封藏之本，精之处也；其华在发，其充在骨，为阴中之少阴，通于冬气。肝者，罢极之本，魂之居也；其华在爪，其充在筋，以生血气，其味酸，其色苍，此为阳中之少阳，通于春气。脾者，仓廪之本，营之居也；其华在唇四白，其充在肌，此至阴之类，通于土气。胃、大肠、小肠、三焦、膀胱，名曰器，能化糟粕，转味而出入者也。"

In the chapter of *Six Sections of Discussion on Zang Xiang* in *Plain Questions*, it's stated in detail that "The heart is the root of life and the house of *shen* (spirit). The heart, which pertains to *taiyang* within *yang* and threads through *xiaqi* (summer-*qi*), manifests its *hua* (luster) on the face and replenishes the blood vessels. The lung, which is the base of *qi* and the dwelling of *po* (soul), manifests its *hua* (luster) on body hair and suffuses the skin. It pertains to *taiyin* within *yang* and threads through *qiuqi* (autumn-*qi*). Being the root of storage and the house of *jing* (essence), the kidney governs dormancy. It manifests its *hua* (luster) on the hair and suffuses the bones, pertaining to *shaoyin* within *yin* and threading through *dongqi* (winter-*qi*). As the foundation of *baji* (enduring exhaustion) and the dwelling of *hun* (spirit), the liver manifests its *hua* (luster) on the fingernails and suffuses the *jin* (sinews). Other features include its generating blood with a sour taste and a dark color, pertaining to *shaoyang* within *yang*, and threading through *chunqi* (spring-*qi*). The spleen, serves as the source of granary supply and the dwelling of nutrient-*qi*. The spleen manifests its *hua* (luster) on the lips, suffuses the muscles, pertains to supreme yin and threads through earth-*qi*. The stomach, large intestine, small intestine, triple energizer and bladder, are all known as containers, playing a part in transforming the dross, and managing the transformation, absorption and discharge of the flavors."

胆、胃、小肠、大肠、膀胱、三焦合称六腑。在古代，腑又通作"府"字，有府库之意。从功能上来讲，六腑主"受盛和传化水谷"，即接受和容纳食物。六腑吸收水谷精微，排泄糟粕，对食物起消化、吸收、输送、排泄的作用。

The six *fu*-organs are defined as the combination of the gallbladder, stomach, large intestine, small intestine, bladder and triple energizer. In ancient times, the character *fu*(腑) could find its equivalent *fu*(府) which indicated the meaning of storehouse. The six *fu*-organs are responsible for receiving, transporting and transforming of food essence in terms of function, namely receiving and accommodating food. The six *fu*-organs absorb nutrients of water and food and excrete the dross, playing the roles of digestion, absorption, transportation and excretion.

有趣的是,中医给五脏六腑都分配了"官职",取象比类,用社会现象来比喻人体。据《黄帝内经·素问·灵兰秘典论》记载:"心者,君主之官也,神明出焉。肺者,相傅之官,治节出焉。肝者,将军之官,谋虑出焉。胆者,中正之官,决断出焉。膻中者,臣使之官,喜乐出焉。脾胃者,仓廪之官,五味出焉。大肠者,传道之官,变化出焉。小肠者,受盛之官,化物出焉。肾者,作强之官,伎巧出焉。三焦者,决渎之官,水道出焉。膀胱者,州都之官,津液藏焉。"五脏六腑可谓分工明确,各司其职。

Interestingly enough, TCM distributes the corresponding "official position" to each of the *zang-fu* organs, adopting the analogy of social phenomenon to describe the human body. Records from *Plain Questions* show that "The heart, which governs the five *zang*-organs from which spirit comes out, is akin to a monarch. The lung is just like a prime minister who assists a monarch in governing the respiratory system. The liver, a military general who is in charge of mapping out well-thought-out strategies and presenting foresight. The gallbladder, a judger who is responsible for making decisions and judgments. The pericardium, an ambassador who regulates *qi* activity and passes information of happiness and joy. The spleen and stomach, a granary manager who is responsible for food intake and nutrients transportation which comes in five different flavours. The large intestine, a transportation official who claims responsibility for changing the food residue into excrement. The small intestine, a reception official who bears responsibility for accepting and accommodating nutrients, which assists digestion and absorption.

The kidney, a powerful official who has a big role to play in essence storing and the smarts of keeping vitality in the body. The triple energizer, a dredging official who has been given charge of dredging water passage in the body. The bladder, a reservoir official who stores body fluid and converges water gradually." These *zang-fu* organs have a clear division of work for each performs its functions.

第三篇　中医四大经典

中医四大经典,即《黄帝内经》《难经》《伤寒杂病论》和《神农本草经》。这些医学典籍的问世,标志着中医理论体系的初步形成。

Section 3　Four Great Classics of TCM

The coming out of *Inner Canon of the Yellow Emperor*, *Classic of Medical Difficulties*, *Treatise on Febrile Diseases and Miscellaneous Illnesses* and *Shennong's Classic of Materia Medica*, which are known in TCM as the four great classics, is the symbol for the primary formation of theoretical system of TCM.

第一章 《黄帝内经》

秦汉时期,我国现存最早的医学典籍《黄帝内经》问世。《黄帝内经》又称《内经》,是中国传统医学四大经典之首。相传为黄帝所作,故冠以"黄帝"二字。它总结了春秋战国以来的医学成就和治疗经验,确立了中医独特的理论体系,奠定了中医药学发展的基础。虽然它成书于数千年前,但今天仍被看作是中医界的权威之作,对中医理论的形成以及临床治疗有着重要的指导作用。

Chapter 1   Inner Canon of the Yellow Emperor

Inner Canon of the Yellow Emperor, the earliest medical classic extant in China, was unveiled during the Qin and Han Dynasties. *Inner Canon of the Yellow Emperor*, also known as *Neijing*, comes up at the top of the four TCM classics. According to the ancient Chinese legend, this classic was written by the Yellow Emperor. Hence it was named after the Yellow Emperor. This classic summarizes the medical achievements and treatment experience since the Spring-Autumn Period and Warring States Period, establishing the unique theoretical system of TCM and laying the foundation for the development of TCM. Although it was compiled thousands of years ago, it is still regarded as a magisterial work in this field, playing an important guiding role in the formation of TCM theory and clinical practice.

《黄帝内经》的成书时间至今未定,作者不详,一般认为起源于轩辕黄帝,代代口耳相传,成书于春秋战国时期,非一人所著。相传《黄帝内经》记载的是黄帝和他的大臣岐伯之间展开的对话,以对话、问答的形式论述了人体的生理、病理、诊断、治疗、养生等问题。全书包括《素问》和《灵枢》两部分,共18卷162篇。

《素问》主要阐述中医基本理论，《灵枢》主要论述九针、经络、脏腑、穴位、刺法以及疾病的诊断治疗等。

Nothing definite is known of the author or the date of its publication. It's generally believed that it originated from Emperor Xuanyuan, and was passed down through word of mouth, then was compiled during the Spring-Autumn Period and the Warring States Period by more than one author. This classic work is purported to be a series of conversations between the Yellow Emperor, and his minister, Qi Bo. Through the questions and answers, it expounds physiology, pathology, diagnosis, treatment, health cultivating of the human body, etc. The work consists of two distinct books: *Plain Questions and Spiritual Pivot*, each comprising nine volumes and 81 articles respectively. *Plain Questions* mainly elaborates the basic theories of TCM, while *Spiritual Pivot* mainly introduces the nine needles, meridians and collaterals, *zang-fu* organs, acupoints, acupuncture technique together with disease diagnosis and treatment, etc.

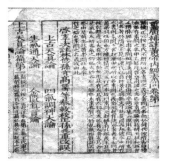

《黄帝内经》
Inner Canon of the Yellow Emperor

该书结合当时其他自然科学的成就，对人体的生理、病理及疾病的诊断，经络，针灸，疾病的症状、治疗和预防进行了全面而系统的阐述，初步奠定了中医的理论基础。《黄帝内经》不仅系统阐述了人与自然的关系，还撷取了哲学、天文、历法、气象、数学、生物、地理等多种学科的研究成果，吸收了包括养生、阴阳、五行、气、天人相应等学说的理念。

Assimilating achievements of other natural sciences at that time, it comprehensively and systematically examines the physiology and pathology of the body, along with diagnostic methods, meridians and collaterals, acupuncture, symptoms, prevention and treatment of diseases, thus laying a foundation for TCM theory. Not only does it offer systematic discourses on the correspondence between man and nature, but it incorporates research results of various disciplines such as philosophy, astronomy, calendar, meteorology, mathematics, biology, geography, etc. It also collected all the experiences and achievements of the methods to maintain good health and longevity, as well as philosophies such as yin-yang, the five elements, qi, correspondence between man and nature, etc.

该书以阴阳学说、五行学说为理论基础,强调了人与自然的密切关系以及人体内部协调统一的整体观念。通过应用阴阳学说、五行学说,《黄帝内经》确立了依据气候和季节条件,地理位置和个人的体质进行辨证治疗的原则,在今天的临床实践中这些治疗原则仍被遵循。几千年来,此书成为中医学必读书籍之一。时至今日,《黄帝内经》中的经典语句仍然有效,为当代中医实践提供了指导。

Based on yin-yang and the five elements theory, it highlights the close relationship between man and nature, and also a holistic and harmonious view of human body. By application of the theories of yin-yang and the five elements, it sets up therapeutic principles of syndrome differentiation treatment based on the climatic and seasonal conditions, geographical localities and individual physical profile. Remarkably, these therapeutic principles are still followed today in clinical practice. It has been one of the must-read books in Chinese medicine for thousands of years. Numerous quotes from this ancient work are still valid today, which provide guidance for the contemporary practice of Chinese medicine.

《黄帝内经》认为养生分为形体保养、形神共养、天人合一三个层次。《黄帝内经》中不乏关于养生的论述:"夫上古圣人之教下也,下皆为之。虚邪贼风,避之有时,恬惔虚无,真气从之,精神内守,病安从来?""春生夏长,秋收冬藏,是气之常也,人亦应之。以一日分为四时,朝则为春,日中为夏,日入为秋,夜半为冬。"《黄帝内经》还强调预防疾病的思想,"是故圣人不治已病治未病,不治已乱治未乱,此之谓也"。养生思想到《黄帝内经》时已经建立起完善的理论体系。

Inner Canon of the Yellow Emperor involves three levels of health cultivation: physical cultivation, physical and mental well-being cultivation and man-nature harmony. There is no lack of ways of cultivating health in this classic, "When ancient Chinese sages enlightened the masses, they advocated the necessity of avoiding *xuxie* (deficiency-evil) and *zeifeng* (thief-wind) in time and keep the mind free from excessive desire. In this way, *zhenqi* (real-*qi*) in the body will be in harmony. If *jingshen* (essence-spirit) remains inside without any loss, disease will find no way to occur." "Spring is the season characterized by resuscitation, summer by growth, autumn by harvest and winter by storage. This is the normal changes of *qi* to which the human body also responds. To divide one day into the four seasons, the morning corresponds to spring, the noon to summer, the evening to autumn and the midnight to winter." *Inner Canon of the Yellow Emperor* also highlights preventative treatment, advocating "paying less attention to the treatment of a disease, but more to the prevention of it". A relatively complete theoretical system of health cultivation is established in *Inner Canon of the Yellow Emperor*.

关于医学教育,《黄帝内经·素问》提出"非其人勿教,非其真勿授,是谓得道"。《黄帝内经》和其他医学典籍曾多次阐述这一思想。《黄帝内经·灵枢·官能》论述九针之法时说"得其人乃传,非其人勿言"。这里的"其人"是指合适的人,即那种不仅具备习医资质,而且能诚心学习、肯为大众服务的人。这些核心理念都是一脉相承的,对中华民族的道德标准、价值取向、伦理规范产生了重要影响。历经数千年,这部中医典籍依旧散发着独特的魅力。

As regards medical education, *Plain Questions* puts forward the idea that "Teaching the right person who is qualified or possesses sincere desire to learn, this is the right way to pass on medical thought and theories." This idea has been stated many times in *Inner Canon of the Yellow Emperor* and other medical works. When expounding the theory of the nine needles in *Spiritual Pivot*, it advocates that "Teach the right person to practice medicine, do not teach or speak too much without consideration." The "right person" here refers to a person who not only has the qualifications of practicing medicine, but also can learn with sincerity to serve the public. These core ideas just come down in a continuous line, which have an important impact on the moral standards, value orientation, and ethical norms of the Chinese nation. During its course of development spanning a couple of millennia, *Inner Canon of the Yellow Emperor* has kept displaying its unique charming in every possible way.

唐朝王冰在《黄帝内经素问注序》中评价这部典籍说:"其文简,其意博,其理奥,其趣深。天地之象分,阴阳之候列,变化之由表,死生之兆彰。"英国著名科学家、历史学家和汉学家李约瑟曾经这样评价《黄帝内经》:"在经历了两千年本土临床实践之后,《黄帝内经》依然保持着它最初成书时中医综合性医学著作的状态,并未发生任何变化。它不仅没有过时或者落后,相反,它还取得了巨大的发展。在它的影响下,中医这个领域名作如林,流派纷呈。如果说中医对世界有过任何贡献的话,那么《黄帝内经》作为一部经典著作应该当之无愧。"

In the *Preface to Explanation of Inner Canon of the Yellow Emperor*: *Plain Questions*, Wang Bing, a medical scholar in the Tang Dynasty, made such comments on this classic, "It is simple in description, profound in meaning, abstruse in theory and deep in taste. It unveils the distinction between heaven and earth, the alternation of yin and yang, the roots of changes and the signs of life and death." Joseph Terence Montgomery Needham, a well-known British scientist, historian and sinologist, also known as Li Yuese in his Chinese name, once gave his comment on this classic, "*Inner Canon of the Yellow Emperor* is in what is described as an original comprehensive state of TCM and still remains unchanged after 2,000 years of indigenous clinical practice. On the contrary, it makes tremendous developments which trigger masterpieces and derived schools in this field. If we can come up with any contribution of TCM, *Inner Canon of the Yellow Emperor* undoubtedly fully deserves this honour."

第二章 《难经》

《黄帝内经》问世之后,另外一部医学典籍《难经》出现。《难经》内容十分丰富,它补充了《黄帝内经》的不足,成为后世指导临床实践的理论基础。

Chapter 2　Classic of Medical Difficulties

After *Inner Canon of the Yellow Emperor*, another classic of medicine, *Classic of Medical Difficulties*, was given birth to the world. This book is rich in content, supplementing what is unaddressed in *Inner Canon of the Yellow Emperor* in many respects, and serving as the theoretical basis for the clinical practice of the latter generations.

《难经》成书约在东汉以前,相传为汉代秦越人(扁鹊)所著,《难经》又名《黄帝八十一难经》,是对《黄帝内经》中81个疑难问题的解答。全书以问答的形式阐明生理、病理、诊断、治疗等各个方面的知识,重点论述了诊脉,以及经络学说和脏腑中的命门、三焦。

Classic of Medical Difficulties was compiled approximately before the Han Dynasty and, according to legend, by Qin Yueren (Bian Que). Alternatively named *Yellow Emperor's Eighty-One Medical Problems*, it deals mainly with the explanations to 81 puzzling medical problems in *Inner Canon of the Yellow Emperor*. A question-answer model is adopted to shed light on the physiology, pathology, diagnostics and therapeutics, especially sphygmology, theory of meridians and collaterals, life-gate and triple energizer of the *zang-fu* organs.

《难经》提出了寸口诊脉法,这和《黄帝内经》提出的全身遍诊法有所不同,为后世普遍推行的寸口诊脉奠定了基础,至今仍指导着中医临床脉诊实践。西汉伟大的史学家司马迁曾对《难经》有如此的评价:"天下至今言脉者,由扁鹊;盖论脉莫精于《难经》。"

Classic of Medical Difficulties puts forward *cunkou* diagnostic method, which is quite different from the whole body diagnostic method proposed in *Inner Canon of the Yellow Emperor*, thus laying the foundation for the common practice of *cunkou* diagnostic method for later generations. *Cunkou* diagnostic method guides the clinical practice of pulse-taking up till now. Sima Qian, a great historian in the Western Han Dynasty, gave an upbeat assessment of this classic: "Among the people who practiced pulse-taking till now, Bian Que made his name fill the world. Among the ancient books and records on pulse, *Classic of Medical Difficulties* rose to the top."

《难经》在《黄帝内经》的基础上有所推阐和发展,成为《黄帝内经》后的又一重要医籍。《难经》出现之后,许多医学院相继成立,各种中医典籍相继涌现,每部典籍都各有所长。

Classic of Medical Difficulties gives further elucidation and development of TCM on the basis of *Inner Canon of the Yellow Emperor* and becomes another important medical book after *Inner Canon of the Yellow Emperor*. After the appearance of *Classic of Medical Difficulties*, many medical schools were established and various classics on medicine were brought into being in succession, each having its strengths.

第三章 《伤寒杂病论》

东汉末年,著名医学家张仲景撰写的《伤寒杂病论》确立了中医辨证论治的基本原则,为我国临床医学的发展铺平了道路。这部典籍被后世誉为"方书之祖",是我国中医历史上第一部临床医学专著。

Chapter 3   Treatise on Febrile Diseases and Miscellaneous Illnesses

Treatise on Febrile Diseases and Miscellaneous Illnesses was compiled by a famous medical expert named Zhang Zhongjing during the late Eastern Han Dynasty. This monumental masterpiece established the fundamental principle for treatment based on syndrome differentiation, thus laying a basis for the development of clinical medicine in later ages. This work is worshiped as "Forefather of Formula", and is regarded as the first clinical classic in the development of TCM.

《伤寒杂病论》总结了东汉之前预防和治疗疾病的丰富经验,全书共 16 卷,包括伤寒和杂病两部分内容。后经西晋医学家王叔和编撰整理分为《伤寒论》和《金匮要略》两部分,前者以外感病为主,共 22 篇,记载 113 个处方,397 条治法,以六经论伤寒,以脏腑论杂病;后者以内伤杂病为主,共 25 篇,记载 40 多种疾病,262 个处方,用脏腑病机理论进行证候分证。外感病和内伤杂病分别论治,表明了中医辨证治疗体系的确立,为以后临床医学的发展奠定了基础。《伤寒杂病论》运用望、闻、问、切四种诊疗方法分析病情,并收选了 300 多个精炼的药方,有很高的使用价值。因此该书也被后人称为"众方之祖"。张仲景因其对中医的杰出贡献,被后世尊称为"医圣"。

In this book the rich experiences on prevention and treatment of diseases before the the Eastern Han Dynasty were summed up. The work is complete in 16 volumes, which comprise two parts, febrile diseases and miscellaneous illnesses. It was later recompiled by Wang shuhe, a medical expert during the Western Jin Dynasty, dividing it into two parts, *Treatise on Febrile Diseases and Synopsis of Golden Chamber*. The former includes 22 articles, recording 113 prescriptions and 397 diagnostic cases. This part puts forward the principles and methods to treat cold-induced febrile diseases arising from exogenous factors by utilizing the six meridian principles to differentiate exogenous febrile diseases and theories of the viscera to differentiate miscellaneous diseases. The latter includes 25 articles, recording 262 prescriptions and more than 40 miscellaneous diseases. This part differentiates patterns with pathogenesis of *zang-fu* diseases. Diagnosis and treatment of cold-induced febrile diseases and miscellaneous diseases are dealt with respectively, indicating the establishment of the system of treatment based on syndrome differentiation in TCM, and laying the groundwork for the development of future clinical medicine. This book analyzes the medical cases by employing four diagnostic methods, and selects more than 300 prescriptions which carry very high value. Hence this book has been known as the "Forefather of Prescriptions" by latter generations. Zhang's remarkable contribution to TCM has earned him the name "Sage of Medicine".

《伤寒杂病论》这部经典是我国医学史上影响力最为深远的不朽著作之一,历代医家无一不把它作为习医之人的必读书目。

As one of the monumental works, this medical classic produces far-reaching impact on the history of Chinese medical science. Physicians of all dynasties without exception view it as a must-read.

第四章 《神农本草经》

《神农本草经》,又名《神农本草》,亦被称作《本草经》或《本经》,成书于东汉,作者不详,是我国现存最早的一部药物学专著。

Chapter 4　Shennong's Classic of Materia Medica

Shennong's Classic of Materia Medica, also known as *Classic on the Herbal* or *The Herbal*, is the earliest book on materia medica extant in China, which was compiled in the Han Dynasty with its authorship unknown.

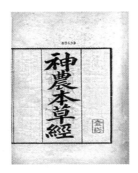 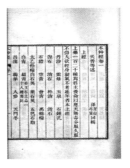

《神农本草经》

Shennong's Classic of Materia Medica

书中载药 365 种,其中植物药 252 种,动物药 67 种,矿物药 46 种。此书详细地记载了每一味药的产地、性质、采集方法和主治的病症等,同时根据药物毒性的大小,将其分为上、中、下三品。上品药无毒,服用可以强身健体;中品药是具有攻治疾病作用的药物;下品药多是治疗疾病的有毒药物。

This classic not only lists 365 medicinal items, comprising 252 herbal plants, 67 animal materials, and 46 minerals, documenting different kinds of herbs and their places of production, properties, collection ways and major functions of every medicine in great detail, but also divides the herbs into three grades according to their toxicity classification: upper, middle, and lower. Medicines of the upper class are nontoxic tonics, performing functions of strengthening and nourishing the body; the middle class ones are drugs with certain therapeutic qualities; and the lower class mainly involves drugs which treat diseases yet are toxic to humans.

该书提出了药物和谐配伍、"四气五味"等药物学理论,认为一个处方应该同时具有"君、臣、佐、使"的药物配伍。此外,该书根据属性将药品分为寒、凉、温、热四性,以及酸、苦、甘、辛、咸五味。该书还提出了"七情和合"学说,即单行、相须、相使、相畏、相恶、相反、相杀七种。

The book sketches the theory of the compatibility of medicinal ingredients as well as "four natures and five flavors of drugs". It holds that a prescription should include at the same time the *jun* (sovereign), *chen* (minister), *zuo* (assistant) and *shi* (messenger) ingredient medicines, and should divide medicines into four natures (cold, cool, warm and heat) and five flavors (sour, bitter, sweet, pungent and salty) according to the properties of drugs. This work also gave expression to the harmony of the seven emotions and established the theory of compatibility of medicinal ingredients—"seven relations", acting singly, mutual reinforcement, mutual assistance, mutual counteraction, mutual inhibition, mutual opposition and mutual suppression.

这些理论为中医开具处方、安全用药及增强治疗效果提供了指导,为后世中药学的形成和发展奠定了理论基础。《神农本草经》作为中华民族的金矿,有待开发利用,造福人民。

All this provides guidance to the production of TCM prescriptions, safe application of TCM drugs and enhancement of the therapeutic effects, thus laying the foundation for the formation and development of TCM pharmaceutical theory. This classic is a gold mine for Chinese nation, which remains to be exploited to benefit millions of people.

第四篇　历代中医名家

Section 4　Renowned TCM Doctors in History

　　几千年来,我国中医史上名家辈出,他们博通岐黄,泽被苍生,著书立说,精勤不倦,开创出蔚为壮观的医林瀚海,为后世的医学发展奠定了坚实的基础。

　　For thousands of years, there is a wealth of renowned doctors coming forth in large numbers in the history of TCM. They attain proficiency in Chinese medicine and make themselves masters in this field so as to exert widely the benefits upon the people. With constant and persistent effort, they write books and set up theories which radiate original ideas to have their voices heard worldwide, stirring spectacular big waves in TCM, and laying solid groundwork for future development of medical science.

第一章　扁鹊

　　扁鹊，原名秦越人，战国时期齐国卢邑（今山东济南）医学家。古人认为，医生治病救人，为病人带来健康，好比带来喜讯的喜鹊，所以古人把那些医德高尚、医术精湛的医生称作"扁鹊"。扁鹊被认为是中国古代医学的先驱，对中医药学的发展有着特殊的贡献，因此被尊为"医祖""中医理论的奠基人"。

Chapter 1　Bian Que

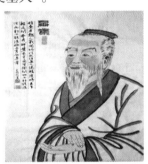

扁鹊像
Portrait of Bian Que

　　Bian Que, originally known as Qin Yueren, was a native of the State of Qi (now Ji'nan, Shandong Province) during the Warring States Period. In ancient China, people believed that doctors went into medicine to cure the sickness, save the patient, and bring health to patients in the same sort of way as *xique* (magpie, a lucky bird) brought some good news to people. Hence the ancients called a doctor with both medical ethics and superb medical skills "Bian Que". Bian Que was widely regarded as a pioneer of ancient medical science of China, and was hailed as the "Forefather of TCM" and "Founder of TCM Theories" due to his great contributions to the development of Chinese medicine.

　　西汉史学家司马迁曾在《史记》中为扁鹊作传。关于扁鹊的史料传说还散见于《战国策》《韩非子》《列子》《韩诗外传》《说苑》等著作中。

　　The story of Bian Que was told in the biography in *Records of the Grand Historian* compiled by historian Sima Qian in the Western Han Dynasty. The historical legends about Bian Que were also scattered in *Strategies of the*

Warring States, *Hanfeizi*, *Liezi*, *Hanshi Waizhuan*, *Garden of Anecdotes*, etc.

扁鹊提出了望、闻、问、切四诊法,为中医诊断治疗奠定了基础。时至今日,四诊法仍被认为是中医诊断的基础。扁鹊精通望诊和脉诊,是中医脉诊法的创始人。《史记》中记载了很多扁鹊治病救人的故事。有一次,扁鹊路过虢国,听说虢国的太子突然死了,扁鹊进宫询问中庶子(太子的侍从官)是否可以看一下太子的尸体,侍从官同意了。扁鹊仔细观察太子的尸体,认为太子没死,而是患了尸厥。他用针灸给太子治疗,并给太子服用了一些中药。不久后,太子果然苏醒了过来。从此人们称扁鹊为起死回生的神医。

Bian Que put forward the four diagnostic methods—inspection, auscultation and olfaction, inquiry, pulse-taking and palpation, laying the foundation for TCM diagnosis and treatment. Even today, the four diagnostic methods remain a foundation for diagnoses in TCM. Being the founder of pulse-taking methods, Bian Que was proficient in inspection and pulse feeling. The book *Records of the Grand Historian* contains countless stories of Bian Que saving lives. Once as he was passing through the State of Guo, he heard about the sudden death of the prince of the state. Bian Que entered the palace and asked an official whether he might observe the body of the prince. The official agreed to his request. After examining the prince carefully, Bian Que concluded that the prince was not dead, but instead suffered a strange and debilitating illness. Bian Que performed acupuncture and gave the prince some herbal medicine. The prince responded to this treatment and regained consciousness immediately. From then on, people believed Bian Que was a highly skilled doctor who could "bring the dying back to life".

传说魏文王曾问扁鹊:"你们家兄弟三人,都精于医术,到底哪一位最好呢?"扁鹊答曰:"长兄最好,中兄次之,我最差。"文王究其原因:"那为什么你名气最大呢?"扁鹊答曰:"长兄治病,是于病情发作之前。因为一般人不知道他事先能除去病因,所以他的名气无人知晓。中兄治病,是于病情初起时。一般人以为他只能治轻微的小病,所以他的名气只及本乡里。而我是治病于病情严重之时。一般人都能看到我在经脉上穿引针管放血、在皮肤上敷药,所以以为我的医术高明,我的名气因此传遍全国。"扁鹊的谦逊审慎由此可见一斑。

According to the legend, once the king asked Bian Que, "You three brothers are all highly-skilled in medicine, who is the best doctor?" Bian Que answered, "The two others are better than me, I am the worst." The king continued to ask, "Then why are you the most famous?" Bian Que replied, "My elder brother gives treatment before the disease arises. Because the ordinary person does not know that he can eradicate the root of disease in advance, so he is unknown to the world. Another brother gives treatment to early illness at the time, most people think that he can only deal with minor ailments, so he's known only to our fellow forks. I give treatment to serious conditions, people observe me perform bloodletting by injecting tubes into vessels or applying medical ointment on the skin, so they look upon me as a great doctor and my fame spreads all over the country." Bian Que exhibited a profound modesty and prudence from this.

良医治病,总是防患于未然。相传扁鹊见蔡桓公,站了一会儿,扁鹊说:"君王,您的皮肤有点小病,不医治的话,恐怕更加严重。"桓侯不理会他,认为医生喜欢给没病的人治病,以此当作功名。过了十天,扁鹊又去拜见桓侯并对桓侯说:"君王,您的病已经到了肌肉里,不医治的话,会更厉害。"桓侯仍然不理睬他。扁鹊走后,桓侯不高兴了。又过了十天,扁鹊再去拜见桓侯,他对桓侯说:"君王,您的病已经到了肠胃里,不医治的话,会更加严重。"桓侯仍不理睬他。过了十天,扁鹊看到桓侯后转身就跑。桓侯特地派人去询问究竟。扁鹊说:"病在皮肤,用汤药洗或者热敷,药力都能达到;病到了肌肉,用针灸也能奏效;病到了肠胃里,用火剂汤也能治好;病到了骨髓里,那是司命所管的事了,医药已经无效。现在他的病已经深入骨髓,所以我也无计可施了。"过了五天,桓侯浑身疼痛,派人寻找扁鹊,扁鹊却已经逃到秦国去了。不出所料,桓侯最终死了。

Good doctors always nip in the bud, preventing the disease from becoming menacing in the very beginning.

Once Bian Que went to the State of Cai and visited the duke of the state, also known as Cai Huangong. Standing for a moment, he told the duke that he had a disease but only in his skin. It would be worse without any treatment. The duke did not listen since he believed that he was fit and considered Bian Que as a physician who just tried to make fame and fortune from others. Ten days later, Bian Que visited the duke again. He told the duke that the disease had gone deeper from the skin to muscle, it would be even worse than before. Duke Cai still turned his back on him and was not happy. After that, Bian Que visited the duke several times and told him each time the disease should be treated in time because it had gone deeper from the muscle to intestines and stomach, and then to bone marrow. But his suggestions were not taken. When he went to see the duke for the last time ten days later, he looked at the duke from afar and rushed out of the palace immediately. When he was asked why he had done this, he said, "When the disease is in the skin, it can be cured by hot compress of medicines; when the disease is in the muscles, it can be cured by acupuncture; when it is in the intestines and stomach, it can be cured by *huoji* soup; but when in the bone marrow, the disease was incurable. It was merely the business of the king of hell. So I'm at my wit's end." Five days later, the duke ached all over and sent for Bian Que, but Bian Que had already fled to the state of Qin. Unsurprisingly, the duke eventually died.

扁鹊不仅精于切脉,诊断准确,而且见多识广。司马迁在《史记》中记载了扁鹊为赵简子治病的故事。在晋昭公统治的时候,赵简子独揽国事。有一次,赵简子生了病,五天不省人事,大夫们都很担忧,于是召见扁鹊诊治。扁鹊进入宫廷,诊察了赵简子的病情就出来了。赵简子的家臣董安于向扁鹊询问病情,扁鹊说:"血脉正常,你担心什么呢!秦穆公也曾经如此,七天后就醒过来了。现在您主人的病和秦穆公相同,不出三天一定痊愈。"过了两天半,赵简子果真醒过来了。

Bian Que was not only known for his proficiency in pulse-taking and accurate diagnosis, but also for his mind of wide scope. According to *Records of the Grand Historian* compiled by Sima Qian, during the reign of Jin

Zhaogong (Duke Zhao of the State of Jin), Zhao Jianzi, known as a *dafu*, had a monopoly on power. Once, Zhao Jianzi fell ill and became unconscious for five days. Other ministers were worried about this and summoned Bian Que for diagnosis. Bian Que entered the palace, examined the disease of Zhao Jianzi and then came out. Dong Anyu, a retainer of Zhao Jianzi, came to inquire Bian Que about the disease. Bian Que responded, "The blood circulation goes smoothly. What are you worrying about? Qin Mugong (the former ruler) used to be like this before. He came to life after seven days. Now the disease of Duke Zhao is the same as that of Qin Mugong. He is bound to recover in no more than three days." After two days and a half, Zhao Jianzi came to himself.

扁鹊行医的足迹遍布很多国家，而且精于内、外、妇、儿、五官等科。作为"经方之父"，扁鹊对早期针灸和药学产生了深远的影响。人们普遍认为中医典籍《难经》是由扁鹊编撰而成。据《汉书》记载，扁鹊曾撰写过两部经典著作：《内经》和《外经》，但都没有保留下来。

Bian Que had left his footprints in many states. He was an expert in many aspects, ranging from internal medicine, surgery, gynecology, pediatrics to ophthalmology and otorhinolaryngology. With the identity of "the Father of Classical Prescription", Bian Que exerted profound influence on early acupuncture and pharmacy. It was widely believed that the TCM classic work *Classic of Medical Difficulties* was compiled by Bian Que. As stated in *History of the Han Dynasty*, Bian Que had compiled two classic works, *Bian Que's Classic of Internal Medicine* and *Bian Que's Classic of External Medicine*, but neither of them was preserved.

司马迁在《史记·扁鹊仓公列传》中记载："扁鹊名闻天下。"他来到邯郸，听说当地尊重妇女，就当起了妇科医生；到了洛阳，听说周都之人敬重老人，就当起了专治耳、目、痹疾的老年病医生；来到咸阳，听说秦地之人关爱儿童，就当起了儿科医生。扁鹊随俗而变，根据各地习俗的不同来调整自己行医的科别，说明他的医术既精湛又全面。

According to *Records of the Grand Historian* compiled by Sima Qian, "Bian Que's name was carried on the wings of fame throughout the country." When he came to Handan and heard that the local people respected women, Bian Que worked as a gynecologist. When he arrived at Luoyang and got to know that the elderly were respected in the capital of Zhou, he served as a geriatric doctor specializing in ear, eye and paralysis diseases. When passing by Xianyang and learning that people in this region of Qin cared for children, he took up his profession as a paediatrician. Bian Que adjusted his medical specialty according to the local custom, which reflected that his medical skills were both comprehensive and eligible.

扁鹊提出了"六不治"的治疗原则。《史记·扁鹊仓公列传》曰:"人之所病,病疾多;而医之所病,病道少。故病有六不治:骄恣不论于理,一不治也;轻身重财,二不治也;衣食不能适,三不治也;阴阳并,脏气不定,四不治也;形羸不能服药,五不治也;信巫不信医,六不治也。"

Bian Que put forward the therapeutic principle of "refusal to treat under six conditions". As recorded in *Records of the Grand Historian*, "What worries the patients most is the prevalence of the disease. While what worries the doctors most is the shortage of effective therapies. Hence the following six kinds of patients will receive no treatment: those who are self-indulgent and unreasonable; those who weigh little on body but too much on possessions; those who fail to adjust diet and clothing accordingly; those with a disorder of yin and yang and a disharmony of *zangqi*; those who are too weak to take medicines; and those who believe in witch doctors rather than doctors."

扁鹊提出的"六不治"的医学思想,对后世医学的发展影响颇大。"信巫不信医,六不治也",彰显了扁鹊的唯物主义思想。"六不治"的医学思想为古代中国的医疗行为和伦理章程提供了框架,成为维护医疗从业者尊严的有力工具。

Bian Que's principle of "refusal to treat under six conditions" is highly influential to the medical development for later generations. Its warning against believing in witch doctors instead of doctors highlights Bian Que's materialist thoughts. A voice of such caution provided a framework of medical behavior and ethical code in ancient China, emerging as a powerful tool to safeguard the dignity of the medical practitioners.

第二章 华佗

华佗,字元化,是东汉末年有名的医学家。华佗是沛国谯县人(今安徽省亳州),约生活于公元2世纪。他擅长外科手术,是世界上第一个发明麻醉剂的医生。他发明的麻沸散由酒和草药混合而成,病人服下后,做手术时就不会感到疼痛。华佗最大的成就在外科手术领域,故而被尊为"外科鼻祖"。据记载,华佗是世界上第一个在外科手术中使用全身麻醉法的医生,他在这一领域的技术比西方早了1600多年。

Chapter 2 Hua Tuo

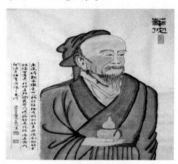

华佗像
Portrait of Hua Tuo

Hua Tuo, courtesy name Yuanhua, was a renowned Chinese physician and surgeon who lived in the late Eastern Han Dynasty. He was born approximately at the beginning of the second century in Qiao County of the Pei State (now Bo County of Anhui Province). Being good at surgery, he was recorded to be the first person to invent *mafeisan* (anesthetic) in the world. The patient who took his *mafeisan*, which was a mixture of wine and herbal medicine, would not feel any pain during the operation. Hua Tuo's greatest achievement was in the field of surgery, and he was thus respected as the "the Founder of Surgery". Hua Tuo was credited with the first recorded use of *mafeisan* during surgery in the world, and his medical skill in this field was more than 1,600 years ahead of that of the west.

华佗也是一位提倡将运动作为保持健康的一种方式的先驱。他创制了一套模仿虎、鹿、熊、猿、鸟五种禽兽姿态的健身操,叫作"五禽戏"。华佗的五禽戏是中华传统文化的瑰宝,不仅具有健身防病之功,还具有丰富的历史文化内涵。正如"流水不腐,户枢不蠹",运动可以让人气行顺畅,防止因瘀血阻滞而致病。《三国志·魏书·华佗传》记载了五禽戏的发明者华佗的一句名言:"人体欲得劳动,但不当使极尔耳。"华佗认为适度运动有利养生。

Hua Tuo is also a pioneer in advocating exercise as a way of maintaining health. He creates *wuqinxi*, literally five animal frolics, featuring a series of animal-imitating movements—tiger, deer, bear, ape, and crane. Being the gem of the traditional Chinese culture, *wuqinxi* (five animals frolics) not only builds up body and prevents disease, but also contains rich historical and cultural connotations. Just as "running water never goes stale and a door hinge never gets worm-eaten", exercise moves *qi* and wards off diseases resulting from blood stasis. As the inventor of *wuqinxi*, Hua Tuo was quoted in *Records of the Three Kingdoms* as saying, "The human body needs physical exercises, but it shouldn't be taken to an extreme." Hua Tuo believes that moderate exercise will be advantageous to health cultivation.

《三国志·魏书·华佗传》记载了"华佗愈躄"的故事,展现了华佗精妙绝伦的针灸技术,多为后人称颂。有人两腿跛足,不能行走,前往华佗处求治。华佗望诊后对病人说:"你针灸、服药已经很多次了。"不等查看完脉象,华佗便让人解开病人的衣服,在背部点穴数十处,每处相距一寸或五寸,穴位纵横倾斜、互不对称。华佗言道:"这些穴位各灸十壮,等到所灸的创口痊愈就可以行走了。"最后,华佗又为病人灸夹脊穴。病人创口痊愈后,行走端直,步态均匀,就像拉直的绳子。

In the book *The History of the Three Kingdoms*, there was a story about Hua Tuo curing a cripple, which demonstrated his fantastic acupuncture techniques and was extolled by later generations. A man who walked with a pronounced limp in both legs came to Hua Tuo for treatment. After inspection of his behaviour, Hua Tuo said, "You have already had excessive acupuncture and medicine." Instead of waiting to finish feeling the patient's pulse, he asked his assistant to take off the patient's clothes. He attacked ten vital points on the patient's back, leaving uneven distance of one *cun* (unit of measurement) or five *cun* vertically and horizontally between each two unsymmetrical points. Hua Tuo then said, "Apply ten moxa cones on each point. You can walk until the wound healed." In the end, the patient had a moxibustion on his *jiaji* points. The patient was responding well to treatment for he could walk with straight back and balanced pace like a straightening rope.

华佗长期在民间行医,足迹遍布安徽、山东、江苏、河南等地,深受百姓的爱戴和敬重。他淡泊名利,不愿为官,多次谢绝朝廷的征召。晚年时期的华佗被一代枭雄曹操征召为其治疗头痛疾病,因为拒绝做曹操的侍医而被杀。

Hua Tuo had long been practicing medicine among the common people, and his footprints covered a great number of places including present-day Anhui, Shandong, Jiangsu, Henan Province, etc. He ranked high in public love and esteem. Being indifferent to fame and wealth, he was unwilling to secure an official position in the court. Several times he had been offered an official position, which he invariably declined. In his late years, he was summoned by Cao Cao, an ambitious and powerful figure during the Three Kingdoms Period, to cure his wind syndrome of the head, and was finally killed by Cao Cao for he rejected to work as his private doctor.

第三章　张仲景

张仲景,名机,字仲景,与华佗一样,也是东汉时期伟大的医学家。因为做过长沙太守,所以后人也称他为张长沙。张仲景幼年因尊崇扁鹊而对医学心生向往,曾师从同乡张伯祖。他确立的辨证论治的中医治疗原则,堪称中医之魂。他对伤寒病颇有研究,所著《伤寒论》《金匮要略》等书籍被奉为中医经典之作。

Chapter 3　Zhang Zhongjing

Another pioneer of the time of Hua Tuo's contemporaries was Zhang Zhongjing, also known by his another name Zhang Ji with a courtesy name Zhongjing, who was born in the Eastern Han Dynasty. Later generations also called him Zhang Changsha for he once worked as the satrap of Changsha (Changsha City, Hunan Province). Since childhood, he was yearning for medical science because he admired Bian Que, and learned medicine from his fellow villager Zhang Bozu. He established the principles of TCM treatment based on syndrome differentiation, which was truly the soul of TCM. He was particularly specialized in the study of cold-induced febrile disease. His books such as *Treatise on Febrile Diseases Caused by Cold* and *Synopsis of Golden Chamber* had all the makings of classics of TCM.

张仲景"勤求古训,博采众方",经过长期的努力,他总结出一整套关于伤寒病的病理、诊断、治疗及用药的完整的理论体系。他认为伤寒病从初起到病危,有一个逐渐发展的过程。伤寒病的治疗应因人而异,在不同的阶段,对不同的病人,应当有不同的治疗方法。张仲景一边行医,一边总结自己的临床经验,记录了许多行之有效的方剂,确立了中医关于伤寒病的治疗原则。在多年行医实践的基础上,他撰写了《伤寒杂病论》这部医学专著，书中提出了辨证论治的治疗原则。这位备受推崇的医学家的不朽著作《伤寒病杂论》对历代习医之人来说都是必不可少的，他为中医做出了杰出的贡献，故而被后世誉为"医圣"。

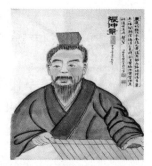

张仲景像
Portrait of Zhang Zhongjing

Zhang Zhongjing learned from classics and predecessors diligently, and collected prescriptions extensively. He labored over the disease for years and summed up a complete theoretical system on pathology, diagnosis, therapy and prescriptions for cold-induced febrile disease. He deemed that cold-induced febrile disease developed gradually from onset till terminal illness. Hence the corresponding treatment should vary with the individual at different phases. Zhang Zhongjing summed up his clinic experience while practicing medicine, recorded numerous effective prescriptions, and established therapeutic principles on cold-induced febrile disease in TCM. Based on years' of practicing experience, he worked out the medical monograph *Treatise on Febrile Diseases and Miscellaneous Illnesses* in which he first proposed the principle of treatment based on syndrome differentiation. The monumental work *Treatise on Febrile Diseases and Miscellaneous Illnesses* compiled by this highly regarded physician is a must for doctors of all generations. He is admired as a "Medical Saint" of Chinese medicine due to his outstanding contributions to TCM.

晋代皇甫谧所撰《针灸甲乙经》记载了"四十眉落"的故事。张仲景遇见了侍中王仲宣，当时王仲宣只有二十几岁。张仲景对他说："你有病，应该及时治疗，否则到四十岁时，你的眉毛就会脱落，眉毛脱落半年后就会死亡。"张仲景还敦促仲宣服用五石汤。王仲宣觉得张仲景的话逆耳不中听，接受了药方却不服药。3天以后，张仲景又见到了王仲宣，问他说："汤药服了没有？"仲宣回答："已经服过了。"张仲景说："从您的面色来看，根本不像服过五石汤的样子，您为什么如此轻贱自己的生命呢？"仲宣仍然避而不答。20年后，仲宣的眉毛果然脱落，眉落后187天便死去了，和张仲景所预料的如出一辙。

In the medical book *A-B Canon of Acupuncture and Moxibustion* by Huangfu Mi in the Western Jin Dynasty, there was a story of "eyebrows shedding at 40 years old". Zhang Zhongjing made the acquaintance of Wang Zhongxuan, an officer in the court, who was only in his twenties at that time. From Wang's look, Zhang Zhongjing identified an insidious disease and told him, "You've got a disease which should be treated as early as possible. Otherwise, your eyebrows will fall off when you are 40 years old. What's worse, half a year later you will die." He urged Wang Zhongxuan to take *wushi* decoction. Zhang Zhongjing's words were harsh to the ear, so Wang Zhongxuan accepted the prescription but refused to take the medicine. Three days later, Zhang Zhongjing met Wang Zhongxuan again and asked, "Have you taken the decoction?" "Yeah, I've taken it." Wang Zhongxuan answered unpleasantly. "There's no hint from your look that you've taken the decoction. Why is your life revealed as cheap?" said Zhang Zhongjing. Wang Zhongxuan still ducked Zhang's question. 20 years later, Zhongxuan's eyebrows shed exactly as expected and died after 187 days, which confirmed the truth of Zhang Zhongjing's conjecture.

张仲景望诊王仲宣,见微知著,这种望诊技术,正是中医治病之奥妙所在。倘若王仲宣听从张仲景的建议服用了五石汤,这场悲剧完全可以避免。

Zhang Zhongjing's inspection diagnosis sees what is coming from one small clue. This is where the secret of TCM treatment lies. Suppose Wang Zhongxuan followed Zhongjing's advice and took *wushi* decoction, the tragedy was entirely avoidable.

据清代汪昂所撰《医方集解》记载,张仲景乃"医方之祖",方剂的发端始于张仲景。后人触类旁通,扩充方剂,然而竟无一人能超越仲景。这或许是前人作法,后人承袭的缘故。创始者难以为用,后起者才容易取得成功。

According to *Collection of Prescriptions with Notes* compiled by Wang Ang in the Qing Dynasty, Zhang

Zhongjing earned the reputation as "the Ancestor of Medical Prescriptions" for medical formula stemmed from him. The later generations single out one thing and bring out this kind of thing by analogy, expanding prescriptions as many as the hairs on an ox. However, Zhang Zhongjing is still unparalleled in his field. Perhaps it's because the predecessors create methods and principles, while the descendants follow accordingly. The rising later generations will come to the top only their founder no longer plays any big roles.

张仲景在《伤寒论》中评论说:"上以疗君亲之疾,下以救贫贱之厄,中以保身长全,以养其生。"他的仁爱之心尽显。张仲景最终成为一代"医圣",是中国历史上最杰出的医学家之一。

Zhang Zhongjing said in his *Treatise on Febrile Diseases Caused by Cold* that "In terms of the higher level, medicine serves for curing diseases of monarch and parents; in terms of the lower level, it functions as the cure for people of humble origin; in terms of the middle level, it plays roles of health cultivation." His kind-heartedness was maximized to the fullest. He finally becomes a "Saint in Medicine" and is one of the most outstanding medical scientists in Chinese history.

第四章 皇甫谧

皇甫谧,字士安,幼名静,后改为谧,西晋安定郡朝那县(今甘肃灵台)人,是汉太尉皇甫嵩的曾孙。

Chapter 4　Huangfu Mi

Huangfu Mi, was first named as Jing at an early age, later changed into Mi with a courtesy name of Shi'an. Being a native of Anding Chaona (now Lingtai of Gansu Province) in the Western Jin Dynasty, he was the great-grandson of Taiwei (supreme government official in charge of military affairs) Huangfu Song in the Han Dynasty.

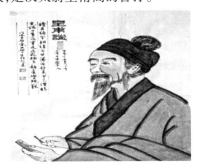

皇甫谧像
Portrait of Huangfu Mi

据《晋书·皇甫谧传》记载,皇甫谧出生后不久,母亲便与世长辞,接着他被过继给叔父,并迁居到新安。他长到二十岁,仍游荡无度,疏于学业。别人还以为他患了痴呆。有一次,他得了瓜果,便进献给叔母任氏。任氏说:"《孝经》中言道:'即便用三牲奉养,依然是不孝。'你如今都已经二十多岁了,眼中不存教化,心中不入大道,没有什么可以让我宽慰的。"任氏感叹道:"昔日孟母三迁,以便培养孟子;曾参特意杀猪,以便取信儿子。难道是我没有选择好居处和邻居,教育有什么失误吗?为什么你冥顽不化至此!勤学修身,自然是你从中得到益处,于我又有什么相干呢?"说完痛哭流涕。皇甫谧深受感动,拜有名的同乡人席坦为师,研习经书。浪子二十始回头,皇甫谧改过自新,勤学苦练。他生活清贫,亲自耕种,经常携带经书务农,博览群书。

According to *Huangfu Mi's Biography in the Book of Jin*, his mother died soon after he was born. Then he was adopted by his uncle, and moved to Xin'an County. At the age of 20, he still neglected his studies. There was no limit to his loafing about the county with nothing to do. In the eyes of others, he was dull-witted. Once he got fruits and presented to his aunt Ren. Ren said, "According to *The Classic of Filial Piety*, it's still unfilial even though three kinds of animals are offered. You are now in your twenties, but are still not on the right track. Nothing else can comfort me." Ren thus exclaimed, "In former days, Mencius' mother moved homes three times to cultivate him, and Zeng Shen killed the pig with special intention to keep promise to his son. Hadn't I selected a good neighbourhood or have I got any fault in education? Why are you such a hard nut? Diligence and self cultivation naturally will benefit you. What can I reap from it?" She then cried and shed bitter tears. Her words touched Huangfu Mi deeply, so he took the famous scholar, Xi Tan, in his village as his teacher to study classics. Huangfu Mi returned to the fold at the age of 20. He turned over a new leaf by studying diligently and training hard. He held simplicity in food and clothes, and grew his own in the farmland. While doing farmwork, he always carried Confucian classics with him. In this way he gained the breadth of reading.

谧母泣教,皇甫谧最终幡然醒悟。从那时起,他立志求学,手不释卷,最终成为举世闻名的文学家、史学家和医学家。这真是应了那句俗话:"浪子回头金不换。"

Huangfu Mi's mother (aunt Ren) gave instructions with tears. Finally her awakening words touched him to repent his actions. From that moment on, Huangfu Mi was resolved to pursue knowledge and finally became a world-famous writer, historian and medical scientist. Just like the old saying goes: "A prodigal who returns is more precious than gold."

皇甫谧40岁时,不幸得了风症,半身麻木,右腿肌肉萎缩。错服寒食散后又引发了药物中毒,全身发热,病情日益严重。寒冬时节,他尚须袒露身体、服食冰雪,到了夏天,则受苦更多:咳嗽、气喘、浮肿和四肢沉重等症状接踵而至,他时刻处于危急之中。病痛的折磨考验着他的意志,求生的欲望又促使他潜心钻研医学典籍,而针灸对于风症的疗效使他对针灸的兴趣日益浓厚,于是他一边研读针灸文献,一边给自己治疗。最终皇甫谧著作等身,在医学方面负有盛名,被誉为"针灸鼻祖"。

At the age of 40, unfortunately, he had a wind-syndrome with symptoms of hemianesthesia and myophagism in his right leg. After mistakenly taking the *hanshisan* (powder medicine for wind-syndrome), which gave rise to drug poisoning, he felt all hot and had been taken worse. During the bitter cold winter time, he had no choice but to leave his body uncovered, eat ice and snow to soothe the body heat. During the summer, he suffered more: Symptoms such as cough, asthma, edema, and heaviness in the limbs came one after another. He remained in a critical condition at any time. The sufferings tested his willpower, and the urge to survive drove him on. So he began to steep himself in medical classics. The efficacy of acupuncture on his wind syndrome fueled his keen interest in acupuncture. He then waded through acupuncture literature, and prolonged illness made himself his own doctor. He eventually achieved celebrity in medical science as a prolific writer, and was extolled as the "Founder of Acupuncture and Moxibustion".

皇甫谧总结了晋代以前中国在针灸方面的成就,撰成《针灸甲乙经》一书。这本不朽的著作共12卷,128篇,涵盖脏腑、经络、腧穴、病机、诊断、治疗、禁忌等内容。该书阐述了经络理论,统一了针灸穴位、名称、取穴法,记载了全身腧穴349个,较《黄帝内经》所记载的穴位增加了189个,建立了较为完整的针灸理论体系,是我国现存最早的一部针灸学专著,也是针灸史上最具影响力的作品之一,为针灸和中国医药产业的发展做出了不可磨灭的贡献,对后世针灸医学的发展有着很大的影响。本书早已流传国外,一度是中外学习针灸的教本,是中医学宝库中的珍品。

Huangfu Mi compiled the medical work *A-B Canon of Acupuncture and Moxibustion* which was a sum-up of China's achievements on acupuncture and moxibustion before the Jin Dynasty (265 A.D.–420 A.D.). This immortal work consists of 12 volumes with 128 chapters, covering *zang-fu* organs, meridian and collateral system, acupuncture points, pathogenesis, diagnosis, treatment, taboos and more. It expounds meridian and collateral theory, unifies acupuncture points, names of acupoints and acupoints selection method, records 349 names of acupuncture points all over the body, 189 more compared with the number recorded in *Inner Canon of the Yellow Emperor*, all of which set up a relatively complete acupuncture and moxibustion theoretical system. Hailed as the earliest extant work dealing exclusively with acupuncture and moxibustion, it is one of the most influential works in the history of acupuncture and moxibustion which has made an indelible contribution to acupuncture as well as the development of the Chinese medical industry. It exerts great influence on the development of acupuncture and moxibustion in later generations. As a gem in the treasure-house of TCM, this monograph has long been spread abroad and served as the textbook for learning acupuncture and moxibustion at home and abroad.

据《晋书·皇甫谧传》记载,皇甫谧性情沉静,清心寡欲,立下了高洁自守的志向,把著书立说当作己任,自己取号为玄晏先生,故而不出仕做官。他酷爱典籍,到了废寝忘食的地步,人们称他为"书淫"。有人劝他,如此将会损伤精神,皇甫谧回答道:"朝闻道,夕死可矣,况命之修短分定悬天乎!"

According to *Huangfu Mi's Biography in the Book of Jin*, Huangfu Mi was quiet, taking "pure mind with few desires" as his pursuit. He aspired to be noble and unsullied, remaining what he was. His mission in life was to write books and set up theories. Thus he named himself Mr Xuanyan, and refused to secure an official position. He was a glutton for classics, almost to the point of forgetting food and sleep. It was for this reason that people called him "Book Addicts". Once he was advised to reduce his commitment for it would enervate his spirit. "If a man has learnt the truth in the morning, he may die willingly in the evening. What's more, one's life span is determined by heaven!" Huangfu Mi responded.

皇甫谧在《针灸甲乙经序》中说："夫受先人之体，有八尺之躯，而不知医事，此所谓游魂耳！若不精通于医道，虽有忠孝之心，仁慈之性，君父危困，赤子涂地，无以济之。此固圣贤所以精思极论尽其理也。由此言之。焉可忽乎？"医道至重，关乎天下民生。这也是后人反复引用皇甫谧这段名言的原因。

As Huangfu Mi stated in *Preface to the A-B Canon of Acupuncture and Moxibustion*, "Our bodies, down to every hair and shred of skin, are received from our parents. A man of flesh and blood actually knows little about medical science despite being eight-feet tall. Isn't that what some people describe as the living dead with indecisive mind? Suppose one is not proficient in medical knowledge, he will definitely fail to aid his monarch, parents and other people who plunged into an abyss of misery when necessary even though he owns loyalty and filial piety. That's why the sages stretch resources to the limit to explore medical knowledge. Medical science, in this sense, can not be ignored." Art of healing is of prime importance for it is vital for people's livelihood. That's why people in later generations repeatedly quoted this excerpt of Huangfu Mi.

第五章　葛洪

葛洪,字稚川,自号"抱朴子",东晋丹阳郡(今江苏句容)人,我国古代杰出的医药学家、炼丹家和道教学者。他不仅发展了道教理论,而且在医学、音乐及文学等方面做出了巨大的贡献。他在中医和科学史上享有很高的地位。

Chapter 5　Ge Hong

Ge Hong, also known as "Baopuzi" with a courtesy name Zhichuan, was from Danyang County (now Jurong County in Jiangsu Province) of the Eastern Jin Dynasty. As an outstanding physician, alchemists and Taoist scholar in ancient China, he not only developed the theory of Taoism but also made great contribution to medicine, music, literature, etc. Ge Hong enjoys a high status in the history of Chinese medicine and science.

葛洪之祖葛奚在三国时期的吴国历任"大鸿胪"等要职,后被皇帝孙皓毒酒赐死。其父葛悌曾任邵陵太守,葛洪为葛悌第三子,颇受其父宠爱。葛洪13岁时,其父去世,从此家道中落。

Ge Hong' grandfather Ge Xi rose to high office such as "*dahonglu*" (a big official) in the imperial court of the Eastern Wu Kingdom in the Three Kingdoms Period. He was later killed with the poisoned wine by the Emperor Sun Hao. His father Ge Ti used to hold the position of satrap of Shaoling (now in Hunan Province) of the Western Jin Dynasty. As the third son of the family, Ge Hong was highly favored by his father. At the age of 13, his father passed away. After his father's death, the family soon declined.

少年时期的葛洪求知若渴,他"饥寒困瘁,躬执耕稼,承星履草……伐薪卖之,以给纸笔,就营田园处,以柴火写书。"他上山砍柴得来的银钱,几乎全都换成了笔墨纸张,一张纸总是翻来覆去地写,直到再无落笔之处。乡人因而称其为"抱朴之士",他遂以"抱朴子"为号。"不学而求知,犹愿鱼而无网焉;心虽勤而无获矣"是他的治学名言。

Since childhood, Ge Hong had a burning desire for learning. "He tumbled deeper into cold and hunger, cultivated the land, mowed the grass under the starlight, cut the wood and sold them for paper and writing brush, and practiced writing with a piece of charcoal in the fields." Almost all the money he got from chopping firewood on the mountain was changed into pens and ink, and he would always write on a piece of paper over and over again until there was no more room to spare. Thus his fellow villagers called him "Baopu Zhishi" (a scholar who clung to simplicity and authenticity), and he then nicknamed himself "Baopuzi". A famous quote from Ge Hong will suffice to typify his scholarship pursuit: "Reading thousands of volumes is indispensable to a scholar, who expects to obtain knowledge, just as fishing net is indispensable to a fisherman, who expects to catch fish. Good intention alone will bring us no gains."

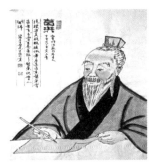

葛洪像
Portrait of Ge Hong

据《晋书·葛洪传》记载,葛洪后来去了广州,在那里,他结识了南海太守鲍玄并拜他为师。鲍玄非常倚重葛洪,不仅将女儿鲍姑嫁给了葛洪,还把平生所学尽数传给了葛洪。

According to *Book of Jin*, Ge Hong later went to Guangzhou where he got acquainted with Bao Xuan, the satrap of Nanhai City, and became a disciple of him. Bao Xuan thought highly of Ge Hong, therefore he not only married his daughter Bao Gu to him, but also unreservedly passed onto him all his knowledge.

到了迟暮之年,葛洪周游于我国南部地区,积累了不少治疗疾病的重要经验。后来,他隐居广东罗浮山,专心著成《肘后备急方》一书。这部大约1700年前的古书为2015年中国药物学家屠呦呦发现青蒿素而获诺贝尔生理学或医学奖提供了灵感。

As he grew into his twilight years, Ge Hong traveled in the southern part of China and accumulated a lot of important experience in treating diseases. Later, he lived in seclusion in Luofu Mountain in Guangdong and concentrated on the book *Handbook of Prescriptions for Emergencies*, a medical book some 1,700 years old, which paved way for the result of Chinese pharmacologist Tu Youyou winning the Nobel Prize in Physiology or Medicine in 2015 as a source of inspiration for her discovery of artemisinin.

据载,葛洪撰有百卷巨著《玉函方》。由于此书过于厚重,不便携带,他就挑选出书中关于临床常见病和急病的内容,另外编撰成《肘后备急方》一书,便于随身携带。此书堪称中医第一部临床急救手册。

It was recorded in the history that Ge Hong compiled another great work *Jade Book of Medicinal Recipes* in 100 volumes. As it was too thick and heavy to carry, he picked out something about clinical common diseases and acute diseases from this book and compiled another book, *Handbook of Prescriptions for Emergencies*, which was easy to carry around. This book has all the makings of the first clinical first-aid manual of TCM.

《肘后备急方》收录的药方皆有"简、便、廉、验"的特点,所以此书很受平民百姓的欢迎。在行医时,葛洪发现很多百姓因无力负担昂贵的药物而放弃治疗,所以他在选用药物时,多选廉价易得之物,一改之前急救药方药物难觅、价格高昂的弊端。

All the prescriptions in the book *Handbook of Prescriptions for Emergencies* had desirable features of "simplicity, convenience, inexpensiveness and effectiveness". Hence the book was very popular among common people. While practicing medicine, Ge Hong found that lots of common people gave up their treatment because they were unable to afford the expensive herbal medicines. Therefore, he tended to select the accessible inexpensive folk herbal medicines, reversing the previous disadvantages of inaccessibility and expensiveness.

《肘后备急方》中的内容包括内科、外科、五官科的知识以及虫兽伤、中毒的治疗方法,所论疾病多以急性疾病为主,为临床急救治疗提供了宝贵的经验。此书相当重视急性传染病,对天花和恙虫病(沙虱)的记载都是世界上最早的。对狂犬病的论述在中国古代医学文献中属于首创。

Handbook of Prescriptions for Emergencies covers knowledge of internal medicine, surgery, ophthalmology and otorhinolaryngology, together with treatment of pathogenic bites by insects or beasts and intoxication. Most of the diseases mentioned in this book are acute illnesses, which provides valuable experiences for clinical emergencies. *Handbook of Prescriptions for Emergencies*, which attaches considerable importance to acute infectious diseases, has the earliest records of smallpox and tsutsugamushi disease (chigger) in the world. The discussions on hydrophobia are a pioneer of China's ancient medical literature.

葛洪集炼丹术之大成,最终撰成中国古代炼丹术的重要著作——《抱朴子内篇》,对后世炼丹术的发展具有重要的意义。葛洪在《抱朴子内篇·仙药》中对许多药用植物的主要产地、形态特征、生长习性、入药部分及治病效果等做了详细的记载和说明,对我国后世医药学的发展产生了巨大的影响。

Ge Hong gathered every aspect and combined some of the best features of alchemy, finally finished the important China's ancient work *The Intrinsic Aspects of Baopuzi* which was of great significance to the development of later alchemy. In his *The Intrinsic Aspects of Baopuzi: Fairy Medicine*, he gave detailed records and illustrations on the main producing area, morphological characteristics, growth habits, medicinal parts and healing effects of many medicinal plants, which vastly affected the development of future generations of medicine.

第六章　孙思邈

孙思邈,京兆华原(今陕西省耀州区)人,是中国医药史上最著名的医学家之一。孙思邈因其杰出的成就被后世尊称为"药王神""药王"。

Chapter 6　Sun Simiao

Sun Simiao, whose birthplace was Huayuan (now Yaozhou District, Shanxi Province), was one of the most famous medical scientists in the history of Chinese medicine. Sun Simiao has been honored by later generations as the "Medicine God" "King of Herb Medicine" for his outstanding achievements.

《旧唐书·孙思邈传》记载孙思邈七岁就学,日诵千余言,有"圣童"之称。长而善谈老庄,兼好释典,通晓百家之说,尤其精于医药。孙思邈淡泊名利,曾三次拒绝隋文帝、唐太宗、唐高宗三朝的征召,成名后过着隐居的生活,专心医学研究。为解救百姓疾苦,他的足迹踏遍了陕西太白山、终南山、山西太行山、河南嵩山、四川峨眉山等山区,采药行医。

According to *Old Book of Tang*: *Biography of Sun Simiao*, Sun Simiao was beginning old-style private school at the age of seven, and was able to recite more than a thousand words in a single day. Thus he had the name of "the Prodigy". When he reached adulthood, he not only enjoyed talking about Lao-Zhuang (Laozi and Zhuangzi) philosophy but also was good at various Chinese classics and literature. He was versed in hundreds schools of thought, particularly proficient in medicine. Sun Simiao refused at least three imperial court positions offered to him by the Emperor Wendi of the Sui Dynasty, and by the Emperors Taizong and Gaozong of the Tang Dynasty since he had reached the state of neglecting fame and fortune. After gaining fame he devoted himself to medical studies and lived in seclusion. In order to relieve the sufferings of the ordinary people, Sun Simiao collected herbs and practiced medicine, expanding his footprints almost every corner of the mountain areas: Mount Taibai and Mount Zhongnan in Shaanxi Province, Mount Taihang in Shanxi Province, Mount Songshan in Henan Province, and Mount Emei in Sichuan Province, etc.

孙思邈倾其一生编纂了《备急千金要方》(简称《千金要方》)和《千金翼方》两部医学经典,各有30卷,合称为《千金方》。这两部典籍共记载6000多个药方,总结了中国自古以来至唐初的医药学成就,堪称中医学发展史上的里程碑。

Sun Simiao devotes all his life to writing out the two TCM classics: *Prescriptions Worth a Thousand Pieces of Gold for Emergencies*, the title usually shortened to *Prescriptions Worth a Thousand Gold*, and *Supplement to Prescriptions Worth a Thousand Gold*, which have 30 volumes each on medical practice and are collectively called *Precious Prescriptions for Emergencies*. Both books, which have recorded more than 6,000 prescriptions and summarized China's pre-Tang Dynasty medical achievements, stood out as one of the notable landmarks in the development of Chinese medicine.

在《备急千金要方》序言中,孙思邈自称其博采群经,删繁就简,力求简明扼要,最终撰成一部涵盖30卷的《备急千金要方》。他认为此书虽不能穷尽所有的病源,但是只要留意此书,也能有不小的收获。人的生命最为贵重,尤胜千金。如果书中的药方能救人一命,再大的善行也不过如此,故以"千金"命名此书。

Sun Simiao claims in the preface to *Prescriptions Worth a Thousand Pieces of Gold for Emergencies* that the book with a coverage of 30 volumes finally comes out by extracting piths from many other classics, simplifying them by cutting out the superfluous and making the selected part be concise and to the point. He deems that although this book fails to thoroughly explore the sources of all diseases, one can still reap the benefits if he keeps an eye on it. Human life is the most precious, and is even worth more than a thousand pieces of gold. There is nothing more virtuous than to save one's life with one prescription in this book in the world. Hence this book bears the name of "a thousand pieces of gold".

《备急千金要方》是中国历史上最早的临床医学百科全书,内容涵盖了内科、外科、妇科、儿科等方面的知识,共分233门,合方论达5300余条。《千金翼方》是对《备急千金要方》一书的补充。

As the earliest encyclopedia of clinical medicine in Chinese history, *Prescriptions Worth a Thousand Pieces of Gold for Emergencies* is comprehensive in scope, ranging from internal medicine, surgery to gynecology and pediatrics, etc. There are altogether 233 categories, involving more than 5,300 articles. *Supplement to Prescriptions Worth a Thousand Gold* is a supplement to his early book *Prescriptions Worth a Thousand Pieces of Gold for Emergencies*.

孙思邈关于医学道德方面的观点在中国医学史上十分重要,《备急千金要方》提出了以"精""诚"为核心的医学道德准则。所谓"精"就是医术精湛,所谓"诚"就是医德高尚。"大医精诚"的医德学说,对中医医学伦理体系的发展产生了深远的影响。

Sun Simiao's perspective on medical ethics is of great importance in the history of Chinese medicine. His *Prescriptions Worth a Thousand Pieces of Gold for Emergencies* puts forward the norms of medical ethics with the core of proficiency and sincerity. The superb medical skills are the so-called "proficiency" and medical ethics "sincerity". The theory of "On the Absolute Sincerity of Great Doctors" has a profound impact on the system of medical ethics in TCM.

孙思邈是中国历史上第一个完整论述医德的人。不仅如此,他还是唐朝时期第一个认识到糖尿病患者应该避免饮酒和吃淀粉类食物的人。

Sun Simiao is considered the first to have presented a thorough elaboration of medical ethics in Chinese history. Besides, he was the first to recognize that diabetic patients should avoid consuming alcohol and starchy foods during the Tang Dynasty.

在长期的实践中,孙思邈积累了丰富的养生经验。在《备急千金要方》和《千金翼方》中,均有《养性》《养老》《食治》篇等论述养生的内容。他提倡疾病应以预防为主,在情志方面要少思、少念、少欲、少语、少悲、少怒等;饮食方面要饮食适度,知晓饮食的宜忌。

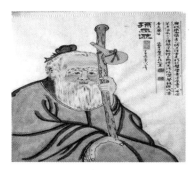

孙思邈像
Portrait of Sun Simiao

In the long-term practice, Sun Simiao accumulates rich experience in health preservation. Both of his two TCM classics, *Prescriptions Worth a Thousand Pieces of Gold for Emergencies*, and *Supplement to Prescriptions Worth a Thousand Gold*, expound the related issues of health preservation in the chapters such as *Nourishing Nature*, *Nourishing Life* and *Dietetic Therapy*. He advocates putting prevention of diseases at the first place, emphasizing "less overthinking, less greed, less desire, less speech, less sorrow, less anger in regulating emotion", "moderate in eating" and "some dos and don'ts of diet".

关于孙思邈的高超医术传说颇多。相传有一次孙思邈回家的时候,遇到四个人抬着一口棺材向野外走去。突然,他看到从棺材里流出几滴鲜血,急忙上前问询。原来棺材里装的是一位孕妇,因为难产,刚死不久。孙思邈言道:"可否开棺一试?我也许能救活她。"孕妇家属知道孙思邈是个医生后,虽然觉得他的话难以置信,但还是决定打开棺材让他试一试。孙思邈为孕妇把脉,发现脉搏还在微弱地跳动着。于是孙思邈在她身上选了一个穴位,扎了一针。不一会儿,这位孕妇竟然苏醒过来了,孩子也呱呱坠地。看到此情此景,众人惊讶不已,孙思邈用针灸救活了一个已被放在棺材里的孕妇,并使该孕妇顺利产子,此乃一针两命矣。

  There are a large amount of legends concerning his superb medical skills. On one occasion, when Sun Simiao was on his way home, he saw four people carrying a coffin to the wilderness for burial. Suddenly he noticed drips of blood from the coffin. So he hurried up for information. Sun Simiao was told that in the coffin lies a pregnant woman who had just died because she failed in delivering a baby. He asked them to put down the coffin at once, saying that he could bring her back to life. Learning that Sun Simiao was a doctor, they opened the coffin in doubt. Sun Simiao felt the woman's pulse and found it beating weakly. He chose an acupoint to give treatment immediately. After a while, the woman came to herself and the baby came out with a cry as well. All went to shock by seeing this. Sun Simiao saved a pregnant woman who had already been placed in the coffin and helped the woman to give birth successfully. This is the anecdote of "saving two lives with just one needle".

  孙思邈擅于治疗各种疑难杂症,救活过很多垂危的病人。有一天,孙思邈的诊所突然抬进来一个病人。病人好几天都没有排小便,肚子胀得快不行了,请求施救。孙思邈为病人进行检查,发现病人小腹绷得像个皮球,病情很严重,服利尿药已经来不及了。孙思邈揣测尿流不出来,大概是尿道不通。这时他留意到一个孩子拿着一根葱管吹着玩,他突然眼前一亮,便拔了一把葱带回诊所。他把葱洗净,去掉根部,小心地从病人的尿道口插进去,一边插入一边往葱管里吹气。终于,充气的葱管把尿道撑开了,尿液立刻流了出来。用一把小葱,孙思邈为病人治好了疑难之症,而孙思邈也因此成为医学史上第一个用导尿术救治病人的医生。这是我国历史上记载最早的人工导尿术。

  Sun Simiao was good at the treatment of intractable diseases and cured many dying patients. One day, a patient was hurriedly carried to Sun Simiao's clinic. The patient asked for help because he had no urine due to a severe abdominal distention for several days. Sun Simiao examined this patient carefully and discovered that the patient's abdomen was swollen like a rubber ball. The condition was so serious that it was too late to take the diuretics. His guess was that the unsmooth urination resulted from the blockage of the urethra. Sun Simiao chanced to notice a child playing with the shallot. An idea suddenly struck him. He pulled a dozen of shallots back to his clinic. He washed the shallots and removed the roots. Then he inserted and at the same time blew into the shallot tube through the patient's urethra carefully. Inflatable shallot finally spread the urethra and the urine immediately flew out. With a handful of shallots, Sun Simiao cured this difficult disease. Sun Simiao became the first one who treated patients by catheterizing. This was the earliest record in China's history of urethral catheterization.

第七章 钱乙

钱乙,北宋著名儿科学家。钱乙通晓各科,尤其精于儿科。他在中国儿科发展史上占有非常重要的地位,是我国医学史上第一个著名的儿科专家。钱乙以"儿科圣手"著称,蜚声中外。

Chapter 7　Qian Yi

Qian Yi, a renowned paediatrician of the Northern Song Dynasty (960 A.D.-1127 A.D.), was proficient in all subjects, especially paediatrics. Being the first established pediatrician in Chinese medical history, he occupies a very important position in the history of paediatrics in China. He is honored as "Sage of Paediatrics" by later generations and enjoys world-wide fame.

钱乙一生著作颇丰,其中包括《伤寒论指微》《婴孺论》《钱氏小儿方》和《小儿药证直诀》,但现在仅存《小儿药证直诀》一书,其他均已遗失。现存儿科专著《小儿药证直诀》是钱乙逝世后,由他的学生阎孝忠将钱乙的理论、临床经验、医案和处方加以搜集整理,于公元1119年编写而成的。这是我国现存的第一部以原本形式保存下来的儿科专著,总结了不同的小儿症状的治疗方法,系统论述了小儿生理、病理特点,治疗上主张以柔润为原则,创制诸多名方,如六味地黄丸等,至今仍为临床所沿用。

Qian Yi wrote much on medicine in his life, including *Detailed Analysis of Treatise on Febrile Diseases*, *Treatise on Babies and Children*, *Treatise on Infants and Children's Diseases* and *Key to Therapeutics for Children's Diseases*. Almost all of these have been lost, with only *Key to Therapeutics for Children's Diseases* remaining. The extant paediatric monograph *Key to Therapeutics for Children's Diseases* was compiled by his student Yan Xiaozhong through collecting and collating Qian's theories, clinical experience, medical cases, and prescriptions after his death in 1119 A.D.. As the first paediatric work preserved in the original form extant in China, this monograph sums up therapies for different paediatric syndromes and systematically discusses the physiological and pathological characteristics of children. It advocates mild treatment as the principle and creates many famous prescriptions such as Tonic Tablets of Six Ingredients with Rehmannia which is still used for clinical purposes.

据宋代刘跂所著《钱仲阳传》记载,钱乙,字仲阳,祖上乃钱塘人,与吴越王钱镠有宗亲关系。吴越第五代王钱俶归宋后,钱乙的曾祖父钱赟随其北上,居于山东郓州。钱乙之父钱颢是擅长用针的医生,然嗜酒好游,一日竟隐姓埋名,东游海上,再不复返。钱乙3岁时,母亲早亡。他的姑母嫁与吕姓的医生,吕先生怜悯钱乙孤幼,将其收为养子。钱乙稍长读书,跟随吕先生习医。姑母临死前才把身世告诉他。钱乙痛哭,请求寻父,往返共五六次,才找到父亲安身之处。几年后,钱乙接父返乡。这时钱乙已经三十多岁了。乡人都为他的孝心所惊叹,感慨落泪,很多人赋诗咏其事。

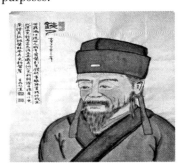

钱乙像
Portrait of Qian Yi

According to *Biography of Qian Zhongyang* written by Liu Qi in the Song Dynasty, Qian Yi, courtesy name Zhongyang, claimed Qiantang (now Hangzhou City, Zhejiang Province) ancestry and clan relations with Qian Liu, the ruler of the State of Wuyue. After Qian Chu, the fifth generation of Wuyue State, fell into state hands of the Song Dynasty, Qian Yun, great-grandfather of Qian Yi followed Qian Chu north to Yunzhou (now Yuncheng County, Shandong Province). Qian Hao, father of Qian Yi, who was skilled at acupuncture drank to excess and traveled extensively. One day, he unexpectedly concealed his identity and traveled east on the sea, leaving everything behind. When Qian Yi was three, his mother died at an early age. His father's sister married a doctor surnamed Lv and adopted him with mercy. As he grew up, he started to read classics and soon afterward followed uncle Lv to practice medicine. During her final hour, his aunt told him about his origins. Qian Yi cried bitterly and requested to look for his father. After going back and forth five or six times, he finally found his father. Several years later, he took his father home. Qian Yi was now in his thirties. His fellow folks were amazed by his filial piety and moved to tears. Many people composed poems, singing praises of his deeds.

钱乙第一次系统地总结了对小儿的辨证施治，使儿科自此发展成为一门独立的学科。他在治学方面最突出的地方，就是"专一为业，垂四十年"。他博采众长，搜集古今所有儿科经方进行研究，在实践中不断提升对小儿生理特点的认识，最终逐步摸索出一整套的治疗方法，如可以通过面部和眼部诊断出小儿的五脏疾病。

Qian Yi is the first one who systematically summarizes treatment of children with syndrome differentiation which enables paediatrics to become an independent subject. What most distinguishes Qian Yi in scholarly research is that he dedicates a total of 40 years to the study of paediatrics. He learns widely from others' strengths, gathering all yesterday's and today's classical paediatric prescriptions for research. Finally a set of treatment methods have been gradually found by means of continuous improvement of the understanding of the physiological characteristics of children in practice. For example, he can diagnose the diseases of five-*zang* organs from eyes and faces of children.

钱乙所撰《小儿药证直诀》一书，最早记载了麻疹、百日咳的治疗方法，也最早记载了从皮疹的特征来鉴别天花、麻疹和水痘，还创立了我国最早的儿科病历。自此书问世后，儿科逐渐发展成为一门独立的学科，因此后人因钱乙对儿科的杰出贡献称他为"幼科冠绝一代"。

The earliest written record of therapeutic methods of measles and whooping cough comes from *The Key to Therapeutics of Children's Diseases* compiled by Qian Yi. Also this book can be said to be the earliest identification of smallpox, measles and chicken pox from the characteristics of the rash ever recorded in written Chinese. What's more, this book also creates the earliest paediatric medical records. Since the appearance of this monograph, paediatrics has gradually become an independent discipline. Hence later generations respectfully address Qian Qi as "unparallel pediatrician in his time" due to his remarkable contribution to paediatrics.

第八章 朱震亨

朱震亨,元代著名医学家,世居丹溪之边,故以之为号,世称"丹溪翁"。他是"金元四大家"中集大成者,中国古代十大名医之一。

Chapter 8 Zhu Zhenheng

Zhu Zhenheng, a well-known medical scientist of the Yuan Dynasty, lived near the Danxi River and was honored as "Danxi Weng" (a man of seniority and virtue) by later generations. He epitomizes the thought of "Four Great Medical Scientists of the Jin and Yuan Dynasties", and is one of the ten eminent doctors in ancient China.

据元末明初戴良所著《九灵山房集》第10卷《丹溪翁传》记载,丹溪翁是婺州义乌县人。姓朱,名震亨,字彦修,学医之人尊他为"丹溪翁"。朱丹溪自幼好学,每天能记诵千余字。稍长,朱丹溪跟随乡里的先生研习经书,以备科举考试。后来他听说许谦先生尽得朱熹真传,时下在八华山讲道,又去拜他为师,日渐了解道德性命之说精深博大,于是将其作为主攻方向。有一天,许谦先生对他说:"我卧病已久,非精于医道者,不能将我治愈。你很有天资,肯不肯学医呢?"丹溪因母亲患过脾病,对医学也略知一二,听了先生的话,慨然道:"读书人如能精通一技,就可借此把仁爱之心推及民众,即便不在朝为官,也如同做官一样行仁道了。"于是他抛却举业,一心致力于习医。

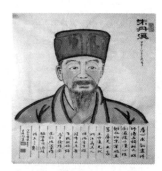

朱丹溪像
Portrait of Zhu Danxi

As stated in the tenth chapter *Biography of Danxi Weng* in *A Collection of Works by Dai Liang* written by Dai Liang in the late Yuan Dynasty, Zhu Danxi, also known as Zhenheng with Zhu as his family name and Yanxiu his courtesy name, was a native of Yiwu County in Wuzhou. Medical practitioners respectfully called him "Danxi Weng". He had eagerness to learn and could recite thousands of words a day since childhood. As he got older, he followed learned seniors in his village to study classics, preparing for the imperial examination. Later he heard that Xu Qian, who had claimed the mantle of Zhu Xi, was preaching in Bahua Mountain. He acknowledged him as teacher and gradually understood the comprehensive and profound theories of morality and human life, which he later made it his specialty. One day, Xu Qian said to him, "I have been confined to bed for long. Only real highly-skilled professional can cure me. You have shown considerable talent for getting what you want, so are you willing to practice medicine?" Zhu Danxi knew medicine slightly for his mother had suffered spleen disease before. On hearing these words, he promised with deep feeling, "One who has the expertise in one speciality can keep a foothold and spread benevolence to the public. Even if he does not rise to prominent positions in the court, he can also practice benevolence like an official." He then gave up the imperial examination and devoted himself to medicine.

朱丹溪著书立说，充分阐明自己的观点，《格致余论》和《局方发挥》是其代表作。他融汇诸家所长，结合自身实践，在医学上不断开创新知，认为人体"阳常有余，阴常不足"，提出"相火论"作为理论依据。治疗上，他主张滋阴降火，后世称其为"滋阴派"。朱丹溪被认为是滋补肾脏和肝脏学说的创始人。他认为阴气精血关乎人们的健康，慢性疾病的主要原因是纵欲过度，建议人们节制欲望，滋养肝肾。

ZhuDanxi writes books and sets up theories to fully clarify his own views. His two representative works are *Treatise on Inquiring the Propensities of Things* and *Elucidation of Dispensary Formulas*. Zhu Danxi integrates other medical schools and combines with his practice, constantly creating something new. He deems that "yang is usually excessive while yin is frequently deficient" and puts forward the "ministerial fire" theory as the theoretical basis.

Therefore, he is inclined to adopt the remedies of nourishing yin and reducing fire in treatment of disease, hence his theory is known as the school of "nourishing yin". Zhu Danxi is considered to be the founder of theory of nourishing kidney and liver. He believes that the yin *qi*, essence and blood is of much concern to people's health. Chronic disease is mainly caused by overindulgence in carnal pleasure without restraint. He suggests people curb unbridled desire and nourish the kidney and liver.

除了《格致余论》和《局方发挥》,朱丹溪还著有《金匮钩玄》《脉因证治》《伤寒辨疑》《本草衍义补遗》《外科精要发挥》等。世上流传的《丹溪心法》《丹溪心法附余》等书乃后人整理朱丹溪的临床经验编撰而成。

Besides *Treatise on Inquiring the Propensities of Things* and *Elucidation of Dispensary Formulas*, Zhu Danxi is also the author of *Mysteries of Synopsis of the Golden Chamber*, *Diagnosis and Treatment Based on Pulse and Etiology*, *Differentiation and Analysis of Exogenous Febrile Disease*, *Supplement to Amplified Materia Medica* and *Elucidation of the Essence of Surgery*, etc. The widely circulated books such as *Danxi's Experiential Therapy* and *Supplement to Danxi's Experiential Therapy* are compiled by later generations based on Zhu Danxi's clinical experience.

朱丹溪在研习《黄帝内经·素问》《难经》等经典著作的基础上,跋涉数省,遍访名师,受业于刘完素的再传弟子罗知悌。正是因为他能谦虚求教且坚持不懈,终成融诸家之长为一体的一代名医。他医德高尚,医术高超,又乐于传医授道,师从他学医的人很多。朱丹溪对后世影响很大。

Based on the studying of the classics such as *Plain Questions* and *Classic of Medical Difficulties*, Zhu Danxi trudged over several provinces, visited famous teachers, and learned from Luo Zhiti, a disciple of the master Liu

Wansu. It is his modesty, willingness to learn and perseverance that eventually paves way for his rising of a great master who integrates strengths of various schools. Not only does he possess noble medical ethics, but his medical skill is superb. He takes delight in imparting his wisdom and knowledge to his disciples, and hence has followers everywhere. Zhu Danxi has a great impact on later generations.

第九章　李时珍

　　李时珍,字东璧,号濒湖山人,出身医学世家,是明朝著名的医药学家。为了编写《本草纲目》这部上百万字的中国医药学巨著,他"读万卷书,行万里路",躬身采集药材,不畏路途艰辛,遍访名山寻药,最终历时27年完成了这部令人难以置信的药物学巨著。这部不朽的巨著集古代本草学之大成,在他逝世以后才得以出版。

Chapter 9　Li Shizhen

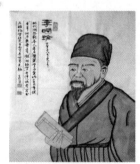

李时珍像
Portrait of Li Shizhen

　　Li Shizhen, also known as "Binghushanren" with a courtesy name Dongbi, one of the most renowned physicians and pharmacologists in the Ming Dynasty, was from a medical family. In order to compile *Compendium of Materia Medica*, a million-word masterpiece of Chinese medicine, he read as many as ten thousand books and traveled as far as ten thousand miles. Despite the arduous journey, he walked around the mountains and rivers of China and risked his life to collect a variety of herbs. His most brilliant achievement was his 27-year effort in writing the incredible masterpiece *Compendium of Materia Medica*, a monumental work published after his death.

　　《本草纲目》集古代本草学之大成,为传统中医提供了重要的参考。这部巨著内容丰富、立论严谨。全书共52卷,共记载了1892种药物,10000多个药方,配有插图1000余幅,内容涉及植物学、动物学、矿物学、物理学、天文学、气象学等方面。这是一部彻底、全面的医学著作,是李时珍对中医药最大的贡献。

Compendium of Materia Medica, which epitomized the pharmaceutical achievements and developments before the 16th century, provides an important reference for traditional Chinese herbalists. This monumental work is rich in content and rigorous in argument. It consists of 52 volumes with 1,892 medicinal herbs, including over 10,000 prescriptions and 1,000 illustrations of medicinal items, covering a wide range of botany, zoology, mineralogy, physics, astronomy, meteorology, etc. This work is a complete and comprehensive medical book ever written in TCM history, which is Li Shizhen's greatest contribution to Chinese medicine.

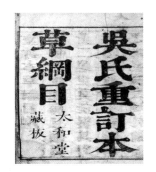 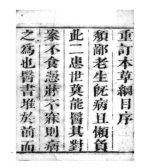 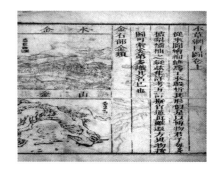

《本草纲目》
Compendium of Materia Medica

《本草纲目》是李时珍倾注了毕生精力的不朽著作,它不仅是中国医学发展史上的光辉成就,也为世界医药学和生物学做出了巨大的贡献。它是世界上第一部对中草药进行分类的专著,对推动中药理论的发展起着开创性的作用,堪称世界医药学的里程碑。这本著作被译成多国文字,对中国乃至世界药物学均有重要贡献和深远影响。19世纪著名生物学家达尔文曾评价《本草纲目》是中国古代医学的百科全书。

Li Shizhen dedicated all his lifetime to this immortal work. It is not only a glorious achievement in the history of Chinese medicine, but also a momentous contribution to the world's medicine and biology. As a milestone masterpiece in world medicine field, *Compendium of Materia Medica* is the first book in the world which scientifically categorizes medicinal herbs. It is a pioneering work that advances TCM pharmaceutical theory. This work has been translated into many languages, and has important contributions and far-reaching influences on pharmacology both in China and all over the world. Charles Robert Darwin, a famous biologist in the 19th century, once evaluated *Compendium of Materia Medica* as the encyclopedia of ancient Chinese medicine.

第十章　叶天士

叶桂,清代著名医家,字天士,号香岩,江苏吴县人。他出身于中医世家,恪守"三人行,必有我师焉"的古训,凡有技高一筹者,他均虚心求教,故而又被后人称为"医痴"。相传叶天士学医曾先后拜师17人,最终名满天下,成为一代宗师,有"国医手"之称。

Chapter 10　Ye Tianshi

Ye Gui, a native of Wu County, Jiangsu Province, also known as "Xiangyan" with a courtesy name Tianshi, was a great medical expert in the Qing Dynasty. Coming from a family of TCM practitioners, he stood by such an ancient precept, "Whenever I walk in the company of two others, I am bound to learn from one of them." He would turn to anyone for advice if one's medical skills remained on top. Thus he earned himself a reputation as "Medicine Science Addicts" by later generations. Ye Tianshi was, according to legend, apprenticed to 17 masters in the medical field successively, and just because of this, he ended up becoming a world-renowned great master. Ye Tianshi enjoyed high prestige and was honored as the "National Medical Master".

叶天士内、外、妇、儿、五官科等无所不通,尤精于温病,是温病学派的奠基人之一。叶天士著有《温热论》,创立了温热病的卫气营血辨证论治,在中国医学史上留下了浓墨重彩的一笔。

Ye Tianshi is proficient in various medical fields, whether it be internal medicine, surgery, gynaecology, paediatrics, ophthalmology or otorhinolaryngology, etc. He is particularly skilled in warm disease treatment and is one of the founders of school of warm disease. *Treatise on Warm Febrile Diseases*, compiled by Ye Tianshi, creates therapies for warm febrile diseases by adopting treatment based on syndrome differentiation system of defensive, *qi*, nutritive and blood, leaving an indelible mark on Chinese medical history.

《温热论》由叶天士的弟子根据其口授编撰而成，书中首次阐明了温病的病因、诊断、治法、传变规律及传播途径，明确提出"温邪"乃导致温病的主因，从根本上划清了"伤寒"与"温病"的界限，为我国温病学说的发展奠定了理论基础，标志着温病学体系的形成。

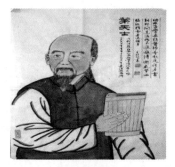

叶天士像
Portrait of Ye Tianshi

Treatise on Warm Febrile Diseases, compiled by disciples of Ye Tianshi according to his oral instruction, elucidates for the first time the cause of disease, diagnosis, therapeutic method, change patterns and transmission route of warm disease in China, explicitly proposes that the "pathogenic warmth" is the main cause of warm disease, and fundamentally draws a clear line between "cold-induced febrile disease" and "warm disease", thus providing a theoretical basis for the development of the theory of warm disease and marking the formation of warm disease system.

除了《温热论》，叶天士的其他著述还有《临证指南医案》10卷、《叶案存真》3卷、《幼科要略》2卷以及《未刻本叶氏医案》，均系其弟子和后裔代为整理编撰而成。

Besides *Treatise on Warm Febrile Diseases*, his other works include the ten-volume *Case Records as Guides to Clinical Practice*, the three-volume *An Authentic Collection of the Case Records of Ye Tianshi*, the two-volume *Synopsis of Paediatrics* and *Unprinted Ye's Case Records*. All these works without exception are sorted out and compiled by his disciples and descendants on his behalf.

叶天士对李杲的《脾胃论》加以补充，首创胃阴学说，提出"夫胃为阳明之土，非阴柔不肯协和"，主张养胃阴。他对中风有独到的创见，认为中风的主要病机是"阳化内风"。另外，叶天士还提出了"久病入络"的学术思想。

The theory of stomach-yin, pioneered by Ye Tianshi, is a supplement to Li Gao's *Treatise on Spleen and Stomach*. This theory proposes that "the stomach, which pertains to yang and earth, get into harmony and balance only with the assistance of yin", advocating the nourishment of stomach-yin. His original ideas about apoplexy spawn his view—the major pathogenesis of apoplexy lies in the "hyperactive liver-yang causing endogenous wind". Moreover, Ye Tianshi raises his academic thought of "a long illness impairing the collaterals".

叶天士关于季节性流行病的理论在很大程度上帮助了中国医生应对2003年发生的非典型性肺炎。叶天士明确地定义了能够引起流行病的疾病，这有助于人们找到更好的治疗方法。叶天士还是中国最早发现猩红热的人。因其杰出成就，后人称他为"仲景元化一流人也"。

Ye Tianshi's theories on seasonal febrile diseases greatly helped Chinese doctors today to deal with SARS (Severe Acute Respiratory Syndrome) in 2003. Ye had clearly defined diseases capable of causing an epidemic, which helps people identify better ways to treat them. He had been among the first, back in ancient China, to find scarlet fever. He has been hailed as "Born-Again Zhang Zhongjing" by later generations for his outstanding achievements.

第五篇　望闻问切

春秋战国时期,"医祖"扁鹊在吸收借鉴前人经验的基础上,提出了中医用以诊断疾病的四种基本方法,即望闻问切,奠定了中医诊断和治疗的基础。

Section 5　Four Diagnostic Methods

During the Spring and Autumn Period and the Warring States Period, Bian Que, "Forefather of TCM", drew on the experience of his predecessors and put forward the four diagnostic methods in TCM— inspection, auscultation and olfaction, inquiry, pulse-taking and palpation, thus laying the foundation of TCM diagnosis and treatment.

四诊,即望诊、闻诊、问诊、切诊,指中医用以诊断疾病的四种基本方法。据《丹溪心法》记载:"《黄帝内经·素问》曰:'能和色脉,可以万全。'"根据中医的理论,四种诊断方法必须综合运用,互相参证,才能弄清病情,正确治疗,即所谓的"四诊和参"。

The four diagnostic methods, namely inspection, auscultation and olfaction, inquiry, pulse-taking and palpation, refer to the four basic methods used in diagnosing diseases in TCM. According to *Zhu Danxi's Experience in Practicing Medicine*, "In *Plain Questions*, it's stated that one will never go wrong if he adopts a mix of complexion inspection and pulse taking at the time of diagnosis." According to the theories of TCM, correct diagnosis and proper treatments can be achieved only if a synthesis of these four methods of diagnosis, which complement each other, is employed. In order to fully diagnose a patient's condition, TCM practitioners are expected to purposefully identify meaningful connections from a large amount of information occurring throughout the human body. That is what "comprehensive analysis is made through the information obtained by the four diagnostic methods" means.

第一章　中医诊断学的发展历程

大约三千多年前,《周礼·天官》一书曾载:"以五气、五声、五色眡其死生。"

Chapter 1　The Development of TCM Diagnostics

As recorded in *The Book of Rites* about 3,000 years ago, "The five *qi*, five sounds and five colors of complexion have put out such a wealth of information that doctors can take it largely to make judgments as to whether the patients are in good health or not."

扁鹊善于运用四诊,尤其是脉诊和望诊来诊断疾病。扁鹊奠定了中医的切脉诊断方法。近代历史学家范文澜评价说,扁鹊乃"切脉治病的创始人"。

Bian Que was skilful at choosing the four diagnostic methods to diagnose disease, particularly at pulse feeling and inspection. The foundation stone for the pulse feeling diagnostic method was laid by this legendary figure. He fully deserved the title of "the Founder of Pulse-Taking Method", said Fan Wenlan, a historian of modern times in China.

中医经典著作《黄帝内经》提出了疾病的诊断需要结合内、外因素,正如《黄帝内经·灵枢·本脏》所言:"视其外应,以知其内脏,则知所病矣。"《黄帝内经》论述了望闻问切四种诊断方法,对于望诊中的望色和切脉皆有详尽的描述,在诊断学的方法上奠定了望闻问切四诊法的基础。

Inner Canon of the Yellow Emperor, a classic of TCM, puts forward that the diagnosis of the disease demands a combination of internal and external factors, just as stated in *Spiritual Pivot*, "Inspection of the external manifestations makes it possible to bring insight into the state of the viscera inside the body, thus aiding doctor's verdict." This classic addresses the four diagnostic methods, and inspection of complexion and pulse-taking are described in detail, thus laying the groundwork for the four diagnostic methods.

中医中的脉诊最为神秘。关于脉诊的专著的数量远远超过了其他医学分支。《难经》尤重脉诊,提出"独取寸口"的诊脉方法,对后世产生了极大的影响。

The art of pulse feeling in TCM is a most mysterious subject. The number of treatises on the pulse-taking far outnumbers other branches of medical science. *Classic of Medical Difficulties* weighs a lot in pulse-taking in particular, proposing the pulse-diagnostic method of "taking the *cunkou* pulse alone" which exerts a huge impact on later generations.

史学家司马迁所著《史记·扁鹊仓公列传》记载了西汉著名医学家淳于意创立的诊籍25例,记录了病人的姓名、性别、职业、地址、症状、诊断、治疗、药方等,这是我国现存最早的病史记录。

Records of the Grand Historian compiled by historian Sima Qian, brought together some of the 25 case records created by Chunyu Yi, a renowned physician of the Western Han Dynasty. This was considered the earliest extant medical history record in China to document patient's name, gender, occupation, address, symptoms, diagnosis, treatment, prescriptions, etc.

东汉末年著名医学家张仲景所著《伤寒杂病论》,确立了中医辨证论治的基本原则,这是中医临床治疗的基本原则。《伤寒杂病论》是中国第一部确立辨证论治法则的医学专著。

Treatise on Febrile Diseases and Miscellaneous Illnesses by Zhang Zhongjing, a distinguished physician at the end of the Eastern Han Dynasty, established the fundamental principles for treatment based on syndrome differentiation, which served as the basic clinical principles in TCM. This classic was regarded as the earliest medical monograph which for the first time built up principles for treatment based on syndrome differentiation in China.

西晋著名医学家王叔和整理古代脉学的文献资料，著成《脉经》一书，这是中国现存最早的脉学专著。该书指出由于脉学理论深奥难懂，故而临床的脉诊方法和技术难以把握，稍有差池，就会造成误诊。该书集汉朝以前的脉学成就，归纳了24种脉象，确立了"独取寸口"的脉诊方法的地位。该书被译成多种文字，流传到朝鲜、日本、欧洲等地。

Wang Shuhe, a famous medical expert in the Western Jin Dynasty, sorted out and combed the documents of ancient sphygmology, and finally compiled the *Pulse Classic*, which was the earliest extant classic on sphygmology in China. "The clinical pulse-taking methods and techniques are all slippery concepts which are hard to grasp for the theory of sphygmology is profound and abstruse to comprehend. A slight mistake will give rise to a misdiagnosis," says the book. As a collection of the achievements of sphygmology before the Han Dynasty, this book summarizes 24 kinds of pulse conditions, and establishes the status of pulse-taking diagnosis method of "taking the *cunkou* pulse alone". This book has been translated into many languages and well on its way around such places as North Korea, Japan and Europe.

隋朝巢元方所著《诸病源候论》是我国现存的第一部论述病源和病候诊断的专著，也是第一部由朝廷组织集体编撰的医学著作，系统、科学、详尽地论述了发病因素、疾病的症状和分类。

Treatise on Causes and Symptoms of Diseases by Chao Yuanfang during the Sui Dynasty was the earliest extant monograph on pathogenic symptomatology in China, and also the first masterpiece compiled collectively under the leadership of the royal court, which expounded the pathogenic factors, symptoms and classification of diseases systematically, scientifically and thoroughly.

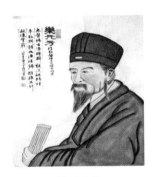

巢元方像

Portrait of Chao Yuanfang

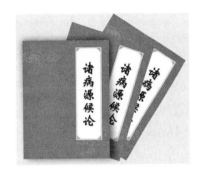

《诸病源候论》

Treatise on Causes and
Symptoms of Diseases

宋金元时期,诊断学方面的著作层出不穷。元代敖氏著有《敖氏伤寒金镜录》,这是我国现存第一部舌诊专著。该书传入日本后,于1654年刊刻出版,并在刻本的基础上形成了多种抄本,对日本的汉方医学诊法产生了深刻的影响。作为舌诊的开山之作,《敖氏伤寒金镜录》奠定了舌诊学的基础,在中国舌诊学史上具有重要的地位。这一时期还有元代医学家危亦林的《世医得效方》和元末明初医学家滑寿的《诊家枢要》问世。

During the Song, Jin, and Yuan Dynasties, the works on diagnostics emerged in an endless stream. Being the earliest extant work on tongue diagnosis in China, *Ao's Golden Mirror Records for Febrile Diseases* by a physician surnamed Ao in the Yuan Dynasty was block-printed and published in 1654 after it had found its way to Japan on the basis of which multiple manuscripts were developed. This book had a profound effect on the diagnostic methods of Chinese medicine in Japan. As a pioneering work of tongue diagnosis, *Ao's Golden Mirror Records for Febrile Diseases* laid the groundwork for tongue diagnosis and had significant standing in the history of tongue diagnosis in China. During this period, *Effective Prescriptions Tested by Physicians for Generations* by Wei Yilin of the Yuan Dynasty and *Essentials for Diagnosticians* by the celebrated physician Hua Shou of the late Yuan and early Ming Periods came out.

明清时期,关于舌诊与脉诊的著作颇丰。如张景岳的《景岳全书》、李时珍的《濒湖脉学》、林之翰的《四诊抉微》和汪宏的《望诊遵经》等。

The Ming and Qing Dynasties were coupled with works on tongue diagnosis and pulse diagnosis being as prolific as before, such as *Jingyue's Complete Works* by Zhang Jingyue and *Binhu's Sphygmology* by Li Shizhen in the Ming Dynasty, *The Essentials of Four Diagnostic Methods* by Lin Zhihan and *Rules of Inspection* by Wang Hong during the Qing Dynasty.

第二章　四诊法

一、望诊

望诊是对患者的总体状况、精神状态及各种体征、舌苔、分泌物、排泄物等进行有目的的观察，是从外到内对病人的审视。在医学实践中，诊断始于望诊，以此来收集数据。中医把望诊归纳为望神、望色、望形和望态四种。

Chapter 2　The Four Diagnostic Methods in TCM

1. Inspection

Inspection acts as examining purposefully the overall condition, covering such aspects as the mental state, physical signs, tongue coating, secretions and excretions of the patients, and also functions as a survey of the patients from the outside to the inside. In medical practice, diagnosis begins with data collection through inspection. TCM reduces inspection into four categories: inspection of the spirit and vitality, inspection of complexion, inspection of physique together with inspection of postures and physical movement.

《史记·扁鹊仓公列传》记载了仓公望诊的故事。齐王有位姓黄的妃子，她的兄长黄长卿在家以酒会客，也邀请了仓公，诸位宾客落座后，尚未上食。仓公看到了王后的弟弟宋建，就告诉他："您有病，就在四五天前，您的腰胁疼痛，无法俯仰，小便又不通畅。如果不及时治疗，疾病就要侵入肾脏。应当趁它未入侵之时赶快治疗。如今疾病将要侵染肾脏,影响小便,这就是所谓的肾痹之病啊。"宋建说:"是啊。我确实腰脊疼痛。四五天前下起了雨,黄家众女婿看到我家粮仓下面有块方石,就过去搬它,我也想效仿他们,但又无法举起,只好又放下它。傍晚时分,我腰脊疼痛,无法小便,到现在也不见好。"宋建的病缘于喜好搬移重物。仓公之所以得知宋建患病,是望到他的面色,他的太阳穴部位颜色干枯。据此,仓公推测他发病应该在四五天前。仓公立刻熬制温补的汤药让他服下,18天左右他就痊愈了。

仓公重脉,仍擅望诊。仓公淳于意通过望面色,准确地诊断了宋建的疾病,显示了高超的望诊技术。

According to Records of the Grand Historian, Huang Changqing, the brother of an imperial concubine Huang Ji, entertained guests one day, and Cang Gong was among the invited. The meal was still not served after all the guests took their place. At that time Cang Gong saw the queen's brother Song Jian and told him, "You look ill, four or five days ago, you failed to bend or stretch due to pain around your waist and ribs. Moreover, you could not urinate as normal. The disease will invade your kidney and develop into urine obstruction without any timely treatment. This will be the so-called renal obstruction." Song Jian responded, "I did have pain in the waist and spine. While it was raining four or five days ago, Huang's sons-in-law saw a square stone under the wall of my granary and lifted it. I tended to emulate them but failed, so I put it down. At dusk, I had the pain in my waist and spine, and was unable to piss. I don't feel better after that till now." Song Jian's disease stemmed from his desire for holding heavy things. Cang Gong found some clues from the inspection of his dull and withered complexion at the temple, which reflected problems of his waist and kidney. In light of all these, Cang Gong figured out that the disease occurred four or five days ago. Then Cang Gong immediately prescribed warming and tonifying decoction for him to take. 18 days later, he fully recovered.

Chunyu Yi, also known as Cang Gong, was not only proficient in pulse-taking, but skillful in inspection. Record showed that an accurate diagnosis was made by Chunyu Yi through inspection, which displayed his state-of-the-art craftsmanship.

朱丹溪在其《丹溪心法》中讲到："欲知其内者,当以观乎外,诊于外者,斯以知其内,盖有诸内者形诸外。"人体是个有机的整体,牵一发而动全身,身体内部局部的病症,可以通过外部显现出来。朱丹溪的这句名言全面阐释了四诊法在中医中的应用。

Zhu Danxi stated in his medical classic *Zhu Danxi's Experience in Practicing Medicine* that "Inspection of the external manifestations facilitates one to know the internal states while diagnosis of the external manifestations promotes one to know the internal conditions. The reason lies in that the functions of the internal organs often have their external manifestations." Human body is an organic whole. Pulling one hair will affect the whole body. Interior local disease can be detected from exterior manifestations. The quotation from *Zhu Danxi's Experience in Practicing Medicine* serves a full explanation for the application of the four diagnostic methods in TCM.

1. 望神

望诊的第一个层次就是望神。正如《黄帝内经·素问》所载"得神者昌,失神者亡",神是生命活动的表现,支配着整个身体。

(1) Inspection of Spirit and Vitality

The first level of inspection is at the level of spirit and vitality. As stated in *Plain Questions*, "Loss of spirit and vitality leads to death while maintenance of spirit and vitality sustains life." Spirit and vitality are the manifestations of life activities and dominate the whole body.

中医强调神形合一,有形才有神,形健则神旺。如果一个人容光焕发,精神矍铄,能与他人有眼神接触,这个人就被说成精神好。反之,如果一个人行动迟缓,反应木讷,动作不敏捷,这个人就会被认为神气不足。

TCM highlights all-in-ones that combine the spirit and the body. Only a healthy body can keep one vigorous. If a person is hale, hearty and energetic-looking, and can make eye contact with others, in this case, the person is said to have good spirit and vitality. Conversely, if a person is slow, dull in response, heavy in body motion, he will be considered lacking spirit and vitality.

2. 望色

望色,主要是望面部的颜色和光泽。颜色分为五种,即青、赤、黄、白、黑,与身体各器官和各种致病因素相对应,古人称之为五色诊。

(2) Inspection of Complexion

Inspection of complexion is mainly concerned with observing the color and luster of the face. In TCM, there are five basic colors: blue, red, yellow, white and black, which the ancients called the five colors diagnosis, corresponding to the conditions of the organs and various pathogenic factors.

视觉诊断是审视反映在皮肤表面的颜色与内部器官的对应关系:肝对应绿色,脾对应黄色,肺对应白色,肾对应黑色。

Visual diagnosis examines the colors on the surface of the skins associated with the internal organs: liver corresponds to green, spleen to yellow, lungs to white, and kidneys to black.

望色还包括观察舌体和舌苔两个方面的变化。舌苔由胃气所生,是舌体上附着的一层绒毛似的苔状物。正常舌象是舌体柔软、活动自如、颜色淡红,舌面有一层薄薄的白苔。

Inspection of complexion also centers on observing the change of the tongue body and the tongue coating which is a layer of fur-like substance covering the surface of the tongue formed by stomach-qi. A soft nimble tongue with lightly red color and a thin white layer is considered a normal healthy tongue.

3. 望形

望形,又称望形体,是指通过观察病人形体的胖瘦、强壮、羸弱、体质形态等来诊断病情。

(3) Inspection of Physique

Inspection of physique is also known as examining a patient's physical build and movement. It refers to the diagnosis of illnesses by observing whether the body is obese or emaciated, strong or weak, in combination with the body build.

形体的强弱与内脏功能的盛衰是一致的,内盛则外强,内衰则外弱。观察病人外在形体的状况可以了解其内在脏腑的虚实和气血的盛衰。

The prosperity and decline of the visceral function are consistent with the strength and weakness of the physical build. The prosperity of the visceral function brings about strong body build, and vice versa. Hence observation of a patient's exterior physical conditions contributes to know the interior deficiency or excess of the internal organs together with the wax and wane of *qi* and blood.

4. 望态

望态,又称望姿态,是指通过观察病人的行动姿态、变化及异常情况等来诊断病情。

(4) Inspection of Postures and Physical Movement

Inspection of postures and physical movement is known as observing quiescent or dynamic movement, postural changes and abnormal movement of a patient.

二、闻诊

闻诊包括听声音和嗅气味。听声音是指听病人的语言、呼吸、呻吟、叹息、咳嗽、打嗝、呕吐、喷嚏、肠鸣等。嗅气味是指嗅病人体内所发出的各种气味以及分泌物和排泄物的气味。

2. Auscultation and Olfaction

Auscultation and olfaction refer to gather information about the patient from listening and smelling. Auscultation covers listening to the sounds of voice, breathing, moaning, sighing, coughing, hiccup, vomit, sneeze and borborygmus, etc. While olfaction involves smelling all kinds of smells emitted from the patient and the odor of the secreta and excreta.

中医认为,肺主气,是发声的动力。肾主纳气,可以帮助肺呼吸并且接受新鲜的空气。通过听声音可以诊察病人体内各脏腑器官的病变以及发声器官的病变。通过闻诊,医生不仅可以得知发音器官的变化,而且可以推断内在器官的病理变化。

TCM holds that the lung governs *qi* and serves as the driving force of voice. The kidney controls reception of *qi* which indicates that the kidney can receive fresh air inhaled by the lung to assist the lung to govern respiration. Hence listening to the sounds of voice can help examine pathological changes of the internal *zang-fu* organs, and the morbid state of vocal organs. By auscultation, the doctor can not only learn about the changes of the phonatory organ, but also infer the pathological changes of the internal organs.

三、问诊

问诊是通过询问病人或其陪同者,了解疾病的发生、发展、治疗经过、现在症状,病人的健康状况、病史、发病经过、发病症状和生活习惯等。《黄帝内经·灵枢·师传》有载:"岐伯曰:'入国问俗,入家问讳,上堂问礼,临病人问所便。'"这说明问诊在四诊中占有重要的地位。

3. Inquiry

Inquiry is a diagnostic method employed to get to know the occurrence, development and previous treatment of disease, present symptoms, health state, medical history, progress and duration of an illness, symptoms, living habits and other things concerning the disease by asking the patient or his or her companion about the disease. As stated in *Spiritual Pivot*, "Qi Bo said that one should inquire the customs when going to a new country; inquire the taboos when paying a visit; inquire the etiquette when reaching the hall and entering the chamber; inquire the patient's living habits and preferences when diagnosing a patient." This shows that inquiry plays a significant role in the four diagnostic methods.

问诊的内容包括患者的一般情况、主诉、现病史、既往史、个人史、家族史和现在症状。

The content of inquiry aims to cover the patient's general condition, chief complaints, history of present illness, anamnesis, personal history and family history together with present symptoms.

一般情况包括患者的姓名、性别、年龄、婚姻状况、民族、职业、籍贯、现住址、工作单位等。

The general condition includes the patient's name, sex, age, marital status, nationality, occupation, native place, current address, work unit, etc.

主诉是指患者感受到的最主要的痛苦或最明显的症状以及本次就诊最主要的原因。

Chief complaints are those associated with the most painful or the most obvious symptoms, signs, the most important reason when the patients see the doctor.

现病史包括起病状况、发病过程、诊治经过和现在症状四个方面。起病状况指的是从发病到出现目前症状的整个过程。发病过程是指从起病到就诊时的病情发展变化过程。诊治经过是指病人患病就诊前所接受过的诊断与治疗情况。现在症状是指病人就诊时所感不适的各种表现,是问诊的主要内容。

The history of present illness embraces four aspects: occurrence of disease, progress of disease, treatment of disease and present symptoms. The occurrence of disease appertains to the whole course of disease from the onset to the present. The progress of disease is something associated with the progress and changes of a disease from the onset to the present time. The treatment of disease means the diagnosis and treatment received by the patient prior to diagnosis. The present symptoms, which serve as the main content of inquiry, unfold the various manifestations of the patient's discomfort at the time of visit.

既往史包括患者平时身体健康状况和既往患病情况。询问既往史有助于辨证论治和临床用药。

Anamnesis embraces health condition in normal times and previous medical history of a patient. The inquiry of anamnesis is helpful for treatment based on syndrome differentiation and clinical administration of medicines.

个人史包括病人的生活经历、平时的饮食起居、精神情志及婚育状况等。生活习惯和饮食偏好直接影响病理状况,这也是个人史被着重强调的原因。家族史包括与病人有血缘关系的直系亲属及与本人生活有密切关系的亲属(如配偶等)的过往和现在的健康状况。由于某些疾病具有传染性和遗传性,因此对家族史的询问不可忽视。

The personal history contains the patient's life experience, daily diet and accommodation, spiritual and emotional state, marital and child-bearing status. The living habits and partiality in diet may directly affect pathological conditions. That is why personal history is highlighted. The family history refers to the health condition in the present and the past of immediate relatives of the patient, and people who are closely related to their life, such as a spouse. Since some diseases are infectious and hereditary, the inquiry of family history should not be neglected.

询问现在症状是指对病人就诊时不适的各种信息进行询问,包括寒热、发汗、疼痛或不适、饮食和食欲、睡眠、大小便的状况等。

Enquiring about present symptoms, which involves the condition of cold and heat, sweating, pain or discomfort, diet and appetite, sleep, urination and defecation, etc.

四、切诊

切诊是通过对病人的某些部位进行触摸、按压来了解疾病的内在变化。切诊包括脉诊和按诊。前者是通过用手诊脉来完成的,而后者是通过用手按压或触摸肌表、胸腹和身体其他部位来检查病理变化。

4. Pulse-Taking and Palpation

Pulse-taking and palpation are performed by feeling, touching or pressing certain parts of the body to understand the internal changes of the disease. The former is done by feeling the pulse, while the latter is carried out by checking skin exposure, chest, abdomen and other parts of the body through pressing and touching by hand for the purpose of examining the pathological changes.

脉诊是中医诊断疾病最常用的方法。脉诊是通过诊察病人的脉搏情况来了解病情及体内脏腑经络、气血阴阳的盛衰变化以及正邪力量的对比状况。对一名有经验的中医师来说，脉象可以揭示病人体内某些机能的失衡。

Pulse-taking, which is an approach by which a TCM practitioner gets to know the condition of the disease, *zang-fu* organs, meridians and collaterals, the wax and wane of *qi*, blood and yin-yang, and comparison of healthy-*qi* and evil-*qi* in the body, serves as the most frequently used method in TCM to diagnose disease. For an experienced TCM practitioner, the condition of the pulse can reflect imbalances that may exist in the patient's body.

清末上海名医毛祥麟在《对山医话》中记述了自己脉诊时亲历的一件事情："余初读《灵》《素》诸书……乃渐通五运六气、阴阳应象之理。每调气度脉，浪决人生死，亦时或有验。……岂知脉理微茫，又有不可臆断者。余有戚某过余斋，形色困惫，询知患咳经月，行动气喘，故来求治。诊其脉至而不定，如火薪然。窃讶其心精已夺，草枯当死。戚固寒士，余以不便明言，特赠二金，惟令安养。时已秋半，及霜寒木落，往探之而病已瘥，细思其故，得毋来诊时日已西沉，行急而咳亦甚，因之气塞脉乱，乃有此象欤！然惟于此而愈不敢自信矣。"

In the late Qing Dynasty in Shanghai, the famous doctor Mao Xianglin presented a detailed account of his own personal experience in the book *Medical Notes When Facing a Mountain*. "When I just started to dip into the medical classics such as *Plain Questions*, *Spiritual Pivot*...I gradually understood five motions, six *qi*, theories of yin-yang and their manifestations. On every occasion I made sure that my breathing was properly tuned, I took the patient's pulse and casually judged life and death of the sufferer. Sometimes my prediction came true....How was I supposed to know the theory of sphygmology were so subtle and profound? As was often the case, I found that I could not make judgement by subjective assumption. One of my relatives who looked drawn and tired once came to me for a cure. Upon inquiry, he had a persistent cough for over a month and breathed hard with every movement.

Examining his pulse, it was unsteady like a flickering flame when dry wood burned. I was in silent shock, assuming that his spirit and essence had been exhausted and his life would come to an end in this withering autumn. I did not tell him face to face for he was actually a poor scholar. I gave him some money, easing his mind so as to take good care of himself. It was already the mid-autumn season at that time. The time had arrived when freezing frost and fallen leaves prevailed. I came to visit him, only to find that he had already been fully recovered. I dwelled on the reason. Could it be that it was due to the time when I felt his pulse? It was at sunset when he came to see me, and his cough aggravated when he hurried on. Thus his *qi* activity was blocked and disorders of his pulse condition were rising, which gave rise to the possibilities of such symptoms and signs. I felt increasingly unable to trust my own judgement at the thought."

脉诊独树一帜,堪称中医诊病的一大特色。这个故事折射出脉诊的精微玄妙。《黄帝内经·素问·脉要精微论》有云:"微妙在脉,不可不察。"而《难经》则用一句话把四诊概括为:"望而知之谓之神,闻而知之谓之圣,问而知之谓之工,切脉而知之谓之巧。"

Pulse-taking develops a school of its own, and has been nothing short of a special feature of TCM diagnosis. This story reflects the subtlety, mystery and profoundness of pulse-taking. *Plain Questions* states that "Pulse-taking is indispensable for all subtleties are reflected by the pulse." *Classic of Medical Difficulties* gives a sum-up of the four diagnostic methods in one sentence: "He who knows the disease by looking is a celestial being; by smelling a great sage; by asking a master craftsman and by pulse-feeling a skillful artisan."

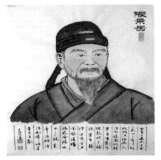

张景岳像
Portrait of Zhang Jingyue

明代医学家张景岳在其所著《景岳全书·传忠录·求本论》中有这样一段

话:"予故曰:'医有慧眼,眼在局外;医有慧心,心在兆前。使果能洞能烛,知几知微,此而曰医。医云乎哉他,无所谓大医王矣!'"这才堪称医学的真谛。

As Zhang Jingyue, a medical expert in the Ming Dynasty, stated in his *Jingyue's Complete Works* that "Therefore, to be a good doctor, one must have an eye for the behind-the-scenes and a mind which perceives signs of future underlying illness. One can be called a real doctor only if he is perceptive of the slightest and knows what is coming from one small clue. Otherwise he is merely an ordinary class of person." This can be the true essence of medical science.

第六篇　中药传奇

中医是涵盖诸多传统医学实践的标签。中医包括中药、针灸、推拿(按摩)、食疗、气功、拔罐、刮痧等治疗方法。正如《黄帝内经·素问》所载："圣人杂合以治,各得其所宜。"中药是中医的重要组成部分,中药主要由植物药、动物药和矿物药组成,其中植物药占绝大多数,使用也更普遍,所以在古代,中药也被称为"本草"。

Section 6　Legends of Chinese Materia Medica

TCM is a label which has a wide coverage of traditional medicine practices. Chinese materia medica, along with acupuncture and moxibustion, *tuina* (massage), food therapy, *qigong*, cupping, *guasha* (spooning) and many other different practices and therapies, make up Traditional Chinese Medicine (TCM). As stated in *Plain Questions*, "Sages adopt a broad repertoire of methods to treat diseases, yet the most suitable one is the best." Key component of TCM is Chinese materia medica, which is composed mainly of plants, animal and mineral ingredients. Among these ingredients, the most commonly used plants account for the majority of TCM treatments. Hence in ancient times, Chinese materia medica was also known as "medical herbs".

第一章　白花蛇舌草

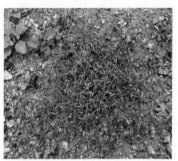 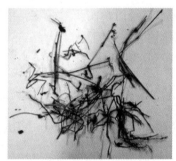

白花蛇舌草
Hedyotis Diffusa

很久以前，有位医术高超的郎中应邀去诊治一位重症病人。这位病人气滞血瘀、胸背疼痛、低热不退、咳吐秽脓，遍请名医皆医治无效。病人因此变得悲观失望，病情更加严重了。

Chapter 1　Hedyotis Diffusa

Long time ago, a highly-skilled doctor was invited to treat a critically ill patient. Concurrency symptoms included qi stagnation and blood stasis, a pain in breast and back, a low fever for a long time together with coughing and vomiting filth and pus. He went everywhere for treatment, tried all sorts of renowned doctors' prescriptions but in vain. Gradually the patient became so pessimistic and discouraged that his condition was getting worse.

家人于是另觅良医。郎中诊断后苦于无方,困乏之际伏案小憩,梦中只见一白衣女子翩然而至,对他言道:"此人乃是贤良之辈,乐善好施,每见捕蛇者,即买下放生,请先生救他一命。"郎中遂向女子讨教良方,女子便道:"且随我来。"

His family then fetched another good doctor. After diagnosis the doctor was suffering from a shortage of appropriate prescriptions. Weary and tired, he couldn't help taking a nap at the table. In his dream, a lady in white flying down from the sky and told him, "This virtuous, kind and generous gentleman's pleasure obtains from his benevolent acts. He always buys snakes from snake catchers and frees them. I beg you to save his life." The doctor then turned to her for effective prescription. "Follow me please", said the lady.

郎中随着白衣女子来到户外,倏忽间,女子飘然而去,郎中低下头,却见女子站立之处一条白花蛇盘旋而卧,口吐开着白花的草。郎中心中正诧异,却被病人家人的脚步声惊醒。于是一同行至梦中所见之处。

Following the lady, the doctor came outdoors. Just seconds later, the lady floated away out of sight. Lowering his head, he found a long-noded pit viper crouching where she just stood. The snake was spitting out clumps of herbs with white flowers. While astonishing, the doctor was woken up by the noise of steps of the patient's families. And they then walked together to the place where the doctor had seen in his dream.

田间果然有许多梦中所见的长势茂盛、开着白花的纤草。郎中旋即采撷一些让病人煎服。服药后,病人感觉疼痛立减,连服数次便痊愈了。

They really found clumps of herbs with white flowers exuberantly grown in the fields. The doctor picked up some of these herbs and then asked the patient to take them in decoction. After taking the medicine, the patient felt a relieved pain immediately. He recovered soon after a consecutive decoction.

激动之余,郎中遍查历代本草,却未查出这纤草的来历,于是美其名曰"白花蛇舌草"。其味微苦、甘,性寒,能清热解毒,利湿通淋,一般用于治疗痈肿疮毒、咽喉肿痛、毒蛇咬伤、热淋涩痛、湿热黄疸。此药药效如神,堪称中药一奇,至今沿用。

With excitement the doctor did a thorough search in the ancient medical classics, but he could not find any traces about the herb. So it was wrapped in a nice-sounding name "hedyotis diffusa". It is slightly bitter, sweet and cold with medicinal efficacies of clearing away heat, eliminating toxicity, removing dampness and relieving stranguria. It is commonly used in the treatment of carbuncle, swelling, sores, toxin, swollen and sore throat, snakebite furuncle, heat stranguria, astringent pain and jaundice with damp-heat pathogen. This herb has been nothing short of a wonder of Chinese medicine and is still used till now for its magic efficacy.

第二章　荜茇

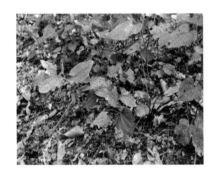 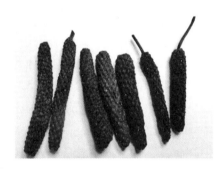

荜茇

Piper Longum

据唐朝李亢撰写的《独异志》记载，唐贞观年间，唐太宗李世民身患痢疾，久治不愈，众太医束手无策，只得下诏求医。

Chapter 2　Piper Longum

As recorded in the book *Duyi Zhi* written by Li Kang in the Tang Dynasty, during the Zhenguan reign period (627 A.D-649 A.D.) of the Tang Dynasty, Li Shimin, the emperor of the Tang Dynasty, had been afflicted with dysentery for a long time and failed to respond to any medical treatment by imperial physicians. Hence the emperor had to send out imperial decree for a cure.

有一位名叫张宝藏的小吏，自己曾患此疾，也是久治不愈，后来他将牛乳和荜茇同煎，饮下后病就痊愈了。听闻这个消息，他就向唐太宗献出此方。

A petty official named Zhang Baozang used to suffer from such intractable long lasting disease, but the decoction of both milk and piper longum soon put him right. On hearing this, he offered the prescription.

唐太宗按此方服药，果然很快就痊愈了。他龙颜大悦，令宰相魏征授予张宝藏五品官衔。魏征愤愤不平，心下不服，就有意为难，超过数月还没有拟旨。后来太宗痢疾复发，仍旧服用张宝藏的药方，药到病除。

After filling this prescription, the emperor recovered soon as expected. He got delighted and ordered the Prime Minister Wei Zheng to rank Zhang Baozang a five-class title. Fuming with indignation, Wei Zheng was very bitter about such overnight success. He was inclined to be hard on Zhang Baozang and did not offer him the rank for months. Later the emperor had dysentery again, and the prescription offered by Zhang Baozang became his magic recipes again.

太宗问起左右："此人献方有功，怎么未见授予官职呢？"魏征有些忐忑，回答道："不知是五品文官还是五品武官，故未授之。"太宗怒斥道："能够治好宰相的病，都会授予三品官衔，现如今治好我的病连五品官衔都不授，难道我还不如你们吗？"随即封张宝藏三品文官，授鸿胪寺卿。

The emperor then asked the officials around, "Zhang Baozang offered the prescription and rendered meritorious service, why don't you give a five-class officer title to him?" These words really made Wei Zheng sweat. He answered, "I was wondering which five-class officer title should be given to him, the civil or the military, so I put it off." The emperor angrily rebuked, "Anyone who can cure the prime minister will be promoted to the rank of a three-class officer. But now Zhang Baozang fails to deserve a five-class title. Am I inferior to all of you?" Zhang Baozang was then given a three-class civil official post, and rose to the rank of Honglusiqing (a high-class official in the Tang Dynasty) in the end.

明朝著名药物学家李时珍认为:"乳煎荜茇,治气痢有效。盖一寒一热,能和阴阳耳。"荜茇味辛、性热,可温中散寒,下气止痛,多用来治疗胃寒呕吐、脘腹疼痛、呃逆和泄泻痢疾。荜茇的用药历史悠久,历代本草多有记载,是中医药历经千年沉淀下来的宝贵财富。

Li Shizhen, an eminent Chinese pharmacologist in the Ming Dynasty, deems that the decoction of both cold-natured milk and warm-natured piper longum is effective in treating *qi* dysentery and helps balance yin and yang. The pungent and warm piper longum with medicinal efficacies of warming the spleen and stomach to dispel cold, and keeping the adverse *qi* flowing downward to relieve pain is often applied for the treatment of abdominal pain due to coldness in stomach, vomiting, hiccups, diarrhea and dysentery. There's a long history of the usage of piper longum as herbal medicine, and Chinese materia medica literatures through the ages have been recording a lot about it. Being a great treasure, piper longum has always been the sedimentary accretion of TCM over thousands of years.

第三章　槟榔

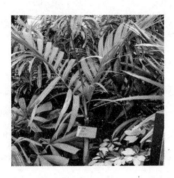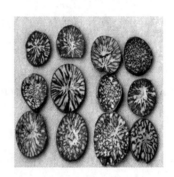

槟榔

Areca Catechu

从前,在五指山下的一个黎寨,住着一位热情纯洁的黎族姑娘博廖(黎语,美丽的意思)。她的歌喉恰似林中的百灵鸟,五指山方圆几百里的后生都想娶她为妻。

Chapter 3　Areca Catechu

Once there lived a pure and enthusiastic girl named Bo Liao (literally, beautiful in Li language) in a stockaded Li Village (an ethnic minority in China) at the foot of Wuzhi Mountain. She sang like a lark in the forest, and all the young men in this area wanted to marry her.

天有不测风云,博廖的母亲身染重疾,只有用五指山顶峰的槟榔作药引才能医治。博廖对慕名前来求婚的后生们说：“我不爱你们的钱财，只会选一个对爱情忠贞不渝的人。谁能把五指山顶峰的槟榔采摘回来，治好我母亲的病，谁就是我要嫁的人。”

A storm might arise from a clear sky. Bo Liao's mother got a critical illness at that time and only the areca catechu at the top of the Wuzhi Mountain could serve as the guiding herb for a better cure. Bo Liao told the young men who came to propose, "I do not love your money, I only want one who will remain unshaken in his loyalty to love. The one who can pick up areca catechu at the summit of the Wuzhi Mountain and cure my mother's disease will be my husband."

五指山就像五根手指，高耸云中，直指苍穹，居于群山之巅，隐于云雾之中。五峰全是悬崖峭壁，凶险异常，从未有人探寻过它的真面目，所以求婚的后生们都望而却步了。

The Wuzhi Mountain was just like five fingers, towering in the clouds, pointing to the sky, squatting at the summit of the mountains and hiding in the clouds. The five peaks were all tremendous cliffs which appeared extremely dangerous, and no one had ever explored its true colors. Therefore, most of the suitors shrank back at the sight.

黎寨青年猎手子黎英勇果敢，深深地爱着博廖姑娘，于是他带上弓箭，义无反顾地走进了人迹罕至的五指山原始丛林。一路上，他不惧林中成群的蚊虫叮咬，不畏蚂蟥的疯狂攻击，日夜兼程，跋山涉水，七天七夜以后终于来到了五指山下。

A brave and courageous hunter of the stockaded Li Village named Zi Li fell in deep love with Bo Liao. With bows and arrows, he came into the inaccessible Wuzhi Mountain virgin forest resolutely. Along the way, he refused to be awed by the mosquito bites in the forest and defied the frenzied attacks of desmodiums. He came across the mountains and waded through rivers, and finally arrived at the foot of the Wuzhi Mountain after seven days and nights.

  子黎沿着山藤和树钩开始攀登。这时一头山豹扑了过来，子黎敏捷地闪过，张弓搭箭，对着山豹连射三箭，射中了山豹的眼睛和喉咙，除掉了山豹。子黎星夜兼程向着五指山的顶峰攀登，眼看就要靠近山顶那唯一的一棵槟榔树，已经可以看到树上红灿灿的槟榔果了，不料一条巨蟒盘在树下，突然张开血盆大口向子黎扑来，要一口吞掉子黎。子黎临危不惧，再次张弓搭箭，射中了巨蟒的眼睛，然后高举大刀，砍死了巨蟒。

  Zi Li began climbing along the mountain vines and tree hooks. At this time a mountain leopard was throwing itself at him. Zi Li dodged agilely, attaching the arrow to the bow and shooting three arrows at the mountain leopard in its eyes and throat. Finally he killed the mountain leopard. Without any hesitation, he climbed the mountain in his full strength all night. At the moment he reached the only betelnut tree at the summit and could see clearly the red areca nuts, Zi Li noticed a giant python lying under the tree. Suddenly the python opened its big mouth and pounced on him, trying to swallow him. Being fearless in the face of peril, Zi Li took out his bow and shot the arrow at the python's eye once again. Then he raised his broadsword and hacked the giant python.

  历经艰辛，子黎终于摘回槟榔果，向心爱的姑娘献上了一份珍贵的礼物。博廖的母亲服药以后很快康复了。两人终成眷属，从此过着男耕女织的幸福生活。

  Going through all the hardships, Zi Li took back the areca catechu. He offered a precious gift to his beloved girl. Bo Liao's mother recovered soon after taking the medicine. Bo Liao and Zi Li finally got married and led a happy life of men ploughing and women weaving.

  槟榔味苦、辛，性温，可驱虫消积，行气利水，多用于治疗肠道寄生虫病、食积气滞、泻痢后重、水肿、脚气肿痛和疟疾。李时珍的《本草纲目》和陶弘景的《名医别录》对此皆有记载。

Being bitter, pungent and warm, areca catechu claims to expel parasites and remove food retention, promote the circulation of *qi* and water as well as activate dieresis. It is chiefly used in the treatment of intestinal parasitic diseases, food retention and *qi* stagnation, dysentery and rectal tenesmus, hydroncus, swelling and pain due to beriberi and edema as well as malaria. Its traces can be found in both *Compendium of Materia Medica* by Li Shizhen and *Separate Records of Famous Physicians* by Tao Hongjing.

第四章 蚕沙

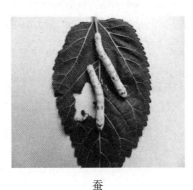
蚕
Silkworm

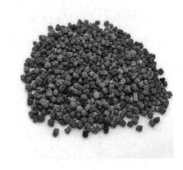
蚕沙
Silkworm Excrement

从前,江南有户人家,父子俩终年在外经商,家里只剩下婆媳二人。婆媳关系紧张,经常拌嘴,所以日子过得并不舒畅。

Chapter 4 Silkworm Excrement

Once upon a time, there lived a family in the regions south of the Yangtze River. All the year round the old man and his son were doing business outside, while the old woman and her daughter-in-law stayed at home. The old woman and her daughter-in-law were on a tight rope and always quarreled with each other. Hence the days did not go smoothly.

有年夏天，媳妇害了火眼，两只眼睛肿胀如桃，几乎无法睁开。媳妇从早到晚悲泣不止。时间久了，眼珠外长出一层白膜，视物不清。

One summer, the daughter-in-law suffered from pinkeye. She cried from morning to night for her eyes had swollen up like peach, and could hardly open. Over time there was a white coat outside her eyeballs which resulted in blurred vision.

因婆媳关系不和，婆婆幸灾乐祸地说："这回你也要用到我了，是否请个郎中开药？"媳妇听出婆婆话中意味，但恐不治会瞎，只好忍气吞声道："既如此，还请婆婆寻医救治。"

Due to their tense relationship, the old lady gloated to her daughter-in-law, "You may need me. Why not call in a doctor for some medicine?" The daughter-in-law knew the meaning behind these words, but she was feared she would go blind. Thus she swallowed humiliation and begged her mother-in-law, "In this case, please fetch a doctor for me."

婆婆请来郎中开具药方，可是并未按方抓药。她心中暗暗诅咒："平日里你待我如此这般，怎么会让你吃这些药？另与你些秽物才是。"

A doctor came and wrote a prescription. However, the old woman did not go to the drug store to fill the prescription. She cursed in her heart, "You usually treat me so bad. How can I give you this medicine? Instead I will give you some filth to eat."

婆婆丢弃了药方，从山坡上捡了些兔子屎，从山洞里掏了点蝙蝠粪。回到家中，她仍愤懑不平，又从蚕铺上添了些蚕屎。她将几种粪便搅拌一通，取了一些煎药，余下的用纸包好。婆婆将煎好的药递给媳妇，口中只道："药已煎好，快服下吧！"媳妇一饮而尽，只觉味道怪异，便问道："这是何种药物，竟无药味儿？"

The old woman threw away the prescription and picked up some excrement of rabbits in the fields and some droppings of bats in the caves. When she got back, she added some dung of silkworms as she went into a sulk again. After having mixed them, she decocted some in the water and kept the rest in a paper bag. Handing the decoction to her daughter-in-law, the old woman said, "It's done. Take it soon." After drinking off the decoction, the daughter-in-law felt its strange taste and asked, "What's this tasteless medicine? It is not like medicine."

婆婆唬她道:"许多草药,只是其中有味好药,此乃'夜明沙',专治眼疾。郎中言道,服此药不仅眼疾可医,便是到了夜晚,看东西也如白日一般。"

The old woman bluffed, "There are many herbs in the soup. Among these herbs there is a so-called 'yemingsha' with remarkable healing properties for eye ailments. The doctor says it will cure your eyes, and will help you see clearly even in the nights as in daytime."

婆婆突然垂怜,媳妇感觉怪异,追问里边还有何物。婆婆低头冥想一番,便道:"还有一味'望月沙'。连服几剂,便能看清月亮中的树木和仙子。"

The daughter-in-law wondered why her mother-in-law took pity on her all of a sudden. She then asked, "Anything else in the soup?" Lowering her head, the old woman thought for a while and answered, "There is also 'wangyuesha' in the soup. Keeping taking this herb, you can see the tree and the fairy lady in the moon."

将信将疑之际,媳妇吃了几天药,谁曾想眼睛慢慢睁开,还真能看见东西了。一日,婆婆外出,媳妇发现了那纸包中的药,闻起来跟吃的药一个味。媳妇仔细一看,是兔子屎、蝙蝠粪和蚕屎,她这才如梦初醒,言道:"婆母欺我太甚,害我不浅!苍天有眼!"她偷偷把纸包藏起,待公公、丈夫回转,再作计较。

Being still doubtful, the daughter-in-law took the herb soup for several days. Who would have thought that she gradually opened her eyes and saw clearly? One day, when the old woman went outside, the daughter-in-law found the paper bag with the so-called herb. It smelled of her herb soup. A closer look suggested that they were excrement of rabbits, bats and silkworms. She became furious with newly-awakened surprise, "My mother-in-law went too far in bullying me and did great harm to me. God has eyes!" She put the paper bag in a hidden place on the sly with the intention of taking revenge when her husband and father-in-law came back.

无巧不成书,媳妇眼疾刚好,婆婆又染上了眼病,比媳妇尤甚。媳妇也如法炮制,假惺惺地请来医生,却用纸包里剩下的三样粪便作药,煎了端与婆婆。

There was no story without coincidences. The old woman was also infected with eye disease which was worse than her daughter-in-law. The daughter-in-law repeated the trick and pretended to fetch a doctor, somewhat falsely. She decocted herb soup for her mother-in-law with the rest of excrements in the paper bag.

婆婆日日服下此"药",几天后,眼疾便愈。一日,她发现盛药的碗底竟有蚕屎,忍不住动怒扔碗:"你这小蹄子,如此猖狂,竟把这等秽物端与我用! 待吾儿回转再作别论!"

The old woman took the "medicine" for several days, and her eyes were perfectly cured. One day, when she had found some silk-worm droppings at the bottom of the bowl, she could not help throwing the bowl in a rage. She scolded, "You are so mean! How dare you give me this! You will be punished when your husband comes back home."

过些时日,父子二人回转家门,婆媳二人争相告状。父子二人经商多年,看出此事中的商机:婆媳二人皆能转危为安,莫非这几种粪便能清热解毒,治疗眼疾?

A few days passed, the old man and his son came back. The old woman and her daughter-in-law attacked each other furiously, competing to recount their respective wrongdoings. The two men ran business for years and spotted business possibilities. Their womenfolk all turned the corner. Could it be that these excrements had the efficacies of clearing away heat and removing toxicity so as to cure eye ailments?

那年夏天,害火眼之人颇多。父子二人干脆就把几种粪便当药送人,结果还真治好了这些人的眼疾。从此以后,婆媳之间再无不睦,一家四口用兔屎、蚕屎、蝙蝠屎合制成药丸和药散,改行售卖眼药,开了家江南最大的眼药铺。

That summer many people suffered from pinkeye. The old man and his son gave the sufferers these excrements as medicine straightforwardly which worked fairly well. Since then, the family was no longer at loggerheads, instead they made pills and powders with the excrements of rabbits, bats and silkworms. Finally they turned to sell medicament for the eyes and ran the largest eye medicine shop in the regions south of the Yangtze River.

蚕沙味甘、辛,性温,能祛风湿,和胃化湿,常用于治疗风湿痹证、吐泻转筋、风疹和湿疹。动物粪便在中医药里并不少见,李时珍的《本草纲目》里有51种动物粪便入药的记载,真可谓物尽其用。唐朝诗人兼作家韩愈在《昌黎先生集·卷十二·进学解》一文中写道:"大木材用作屋梁,小木料当作椽子,各得所用,建成房屋,此乃工匠的技巧。玉屑、朱砂、天麻、青芝、牛尿、马勃、破朽鼓皮,都兼收并蓄,待用无遗,此乃医者的妙用。"蚕沙历来是中医行医者们钟爱的良药。

Silkworm excrement, which claims to expel wind-dampness, relieve rheumatism, harmonize the stomach and resolve dampness, is sweet, pungent and warm. It is often applied for diseases such as rheumatic arthralgia, vomit, diarrhea and cramp, rubella and eczema. Animal wastes are not uncommon in TCM. Up to 51 kinds of animal wastes used as medicine have been documented in *Compendium of Materia Medica* by Li Shizhen, which makes the best use of everything. As stated in *A Collection of Mr Changli* by poet and writer Han Yu from the Tang Dynasty,

"Big timber can be used as roof beams and small ones as rafters for construction of new houses. This is how a skilled craftsman always makes use of whatever he can. Nephrite grains, cinnabar, rhizoma gastrodiae and lucid ganoderma are all precious and costly medicinal materials. Conversely, cow urine, wild fungus, worn-down drum head which has fallen into disrepair, these seemingly useless and worthless ingredients also possess healing power if handled properly. TCM practitioners work miracles when they take in a synthesis of these different kinds of ingredients despite their diverse nature and make the most of things." As a good remedy, silkworm excrement has always been preferred by TCM practitioners.

第五章　车前草

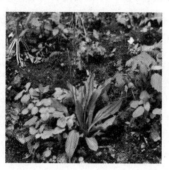 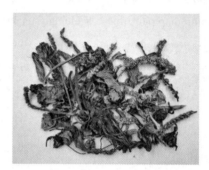

车前草

Plantain

相传有一次，汉朝名将马武带领军队去征讨武陵的羌人。由于地形生疏，马武将军打了败仗，被围困在一个人迹罕至的地方。时值盛夏，又久旱无雨，士兵们找不到粮食，连喝水也变得困难。将士和战马都因缺水得了尿血症，而当地又没有清热利水的药物，将士们个个忧心忡忡。

Chapter 5　Plantain

According to legend, during the Han Dynasty, the famous general Ma Wu led his army to conquer the Qiang people in the Wuling area. Since they were unfamiliar with the terrain, general Ma Wu lost the battle and was besieged in an untraversed region. It was high-summer and the area suffered from a severe drought. The soldiers could see no way out of the situation for they found neither food nor water. The soldiers and the horses all had hematuria due to a water shortage. What was even worse, there was no herb which could reduce heat and excrete water nearby. The soldiers were all laden with anxiety.

这时,一个名叫张勇的马夫发现有几匹患尿血症的战马竟然不治而愈,出于好奇便一寻究竟,他发现地面上有一片猪耳形的野草被战马吃光了。

At this time, a groom named Zhang Yong discovered that several horses which had developed hematuria achieved spontaneous healing. Out of curiosity, he decided to find out the truth. He discovered, on closer inspection, that some pig-ear like grass on the ground had been eaten up by the horses.

张勇决定亲自试服来验证其药效,结果这猪耳形的草竟真的是救星。于是他立刻将此事禀告马武将军。将军闻听喜不自禁,询问此草生于何处。张勇用手指着说:"就在马车前面。"马武哈哈大笑:"这真是天助我也,好个车前草!"当即命令全军吃下此草,果然治愈了尿血症。车前草的名字就这样传开了。

Zhang Yong determined to test the efficacy of the herb in person. It turned out to be that the grass really was a lifesaver. So he told the general this good news immediately. The general asked with overwhelming joy, "Where is the grass?" Zhang Yong pointed his finger at the carriage and said, "It's over there, just in front of the carriage." The general laughed heartily and said, "This is really help from heaven! A magic grass in front of the carriage, indeed!" He ordered the whole army to eat the grass right away. Sure enough, there was hope of a cure. Since then, the name of plantain began to spread.

车前草味甘、性微寒。它的主要功效是利水通淋、渗湿止泻、清肝明目、祛痰。
Being sweet and slightly cold, plantain has the main efficacies of promoting urination, relieving stranguria, excreting dampness, stopping diarrhea, clearing away liver-fire to brighten the eyes and resolving phlegm.

第六章　穿山龙

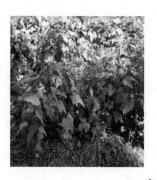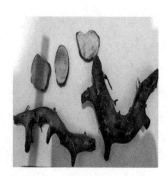

穿山龙
Dioscoreae Nipponicae

很久以前,在长白山一带很多人会得一种怪病,起初是腰酸腿痛,后来就慢慢发展成瘫痪在床。得了这种病,生活就会变得艰辛无比。

Chapter 6　Dioscoreae Nipponicae

Long long ago, many people who lived near the Changbai Mountain suffered from a strange disease which caused pain in waist and legs at first, and then gradually developed into being confined to bed. This illness would mean a harsh and miserable time.

长白山一带虽然地域辽阔,但药铺只有一家,开药铺的是一位老者和他的女儿初夏。老者医术精湛、心地善良,为穷人治病从不收取诊费,当地人都尊他为"老中医"。他的小女儿也颇懂医术,经常同父亲出门采撷草药。

Although Changbai Mountain had a vast area, there was only one herbal medicine shop in this area run by an old man and his young daughter Chu Xia. The highly skilled and kind-hearted old man always helped the poor without any medical fees. So the local people looked up to him as an "old Chinese medicine practitioner". His little girl also knew how to practice medicine and often went to collect herbs with her father.

对于这一带人的怪病,老中医一直甚为苦恼,因为他始终找不到能够治疗这种疾病的草药。每天上门求诊的病人屡受打击,他们存抱希望而来,却屡次失望而归。初夏了解父亲的心事,她暗自下定决心一定要想办法治愈他们。

The old Chinese medicine practitioner was constantly gnawed by the strange disease for he failed to find the cure for it. The patients were hit time and time again by the ineffective treatment. Though each time it seemed hopeful, the results were always disappointed at last. Chu Xia could understand her father's innermost feelings, and she determined to think of ways to heal them.

有一天,初夏背着一个竹筐去龙潭采药,筐里装了一把镰刀和一些食物。听老人们说龙潭是个很凶险的地方,那里经常有野兽出没,黑龙精也住在那里,许多猎人都不敢去冒险。但初夏认为,那里一定有可以治病的珍稀草药,所以就毫不犹豫地出发了。

One day, she headed to Dragon Pond to collect herbs with a bamboo basket which contained a sickle and some food. It was said by the old men that Dragon Pond was extremely dangerous and there were many wild animals, especially a monster called Black Dragon. Many hunters dared not go to Dragon Pond to take risks. However, Chu Xia thought that she could definitely find some rare herbs to cure this disease, and so her adventure was carried out without any hesitation.

跋山涉水，初夏来到了龙潭。她先在山边搭了个草棚,然后她便背着竹筐上山寻药了。初夏遍尝百草，竟无一种适用，不禁心下悲凄。她回至草棚，想起乡亲们瘫痪不能动弹的样子，想起父亲焦虑的神情，难过地哭了。她含着泪水睡着了，梦中有一位黑衣青年来到草棚，初夏惊问："来者何人？意欲何为？"青年人彬彬有礼地作揖言道："我非常敬佩姑娘的胆识，愿助姑娘一臂之力，共同找寻良药。"

Chu Xia came across mountains and waded though rivers, and finally arrived at Dragon Pond. She first built a straw hut by the side of the mountain, settled down, and then immediately climbed the mountain to seek herbs with a bamboo basket on her back without any delay. She tried many herbs, but could not find the right one. Feeling sad, she went back to her straw hut. When the plight of her folks and the anxious looks of her father rose before her, she cried with grief. Then she fell in sleep with tears. A young man in black came into her dream. She was surprised and asked, "Who are you? What do you want?" The young man bowed and said politely, "I admire your bravery, and intend to lend you a hand to find the herb which can cure the disease."

初夏言道："遍寻龙潭，竟无一种适用的草药。"黑衣青年宽慰她："姑娘别急，只管在草棚里等候便是。待天亮后到草棚外面去挖一种带龙鳞的草根即可。"说完，黑衣青年就走了。一转眼天黑了，电闪雷鸣，暴雨将至。初夏从梦中惊醒，定神向外窥探，才发现竟和梦中情境一样。初夏忙冲出草棚，只见天上有一条小黑龙，正往山上撞，每撞一下就落下许多龙鳞，初夏顿时流下了眼泪，不忍再看，转身走进了草棚。不一会儿，天色渐亮，初夏便依梦中黑衣青年的叮嘱，走出草棚。果然，她一出来就看见草棚外面长了许多鱼鳞状的草，初夏意识到这就是那个黑衣青年所说的带龙鳞的草，也就是小黑龙身上的鳞片。她心中异常感动，便含着眼泪挖了满满一筐草根带下山。

"I have searched every corner of Dragon Pond, none of the herbs is useful." said Chu Xia. "Don't worry. You just stay in the straw hut. When the daybreak comes, you go out of the straw hut to dig the root of the grass with the black dragon scales." With these words, the young man left. It was dark in a blink of an eye. The lightning flashed and the thunder rumbled. It was about to rain. The girl woke up and looked outside. It was just like what was it in her dream. She went out and saw a little black dragon in the sky which was striking itself against the hills. With every collision, lots of dragon scales fell down. The girl burst into tears and went back to the straw hut for she could not bear to see that anymore. After a while, when the new day came, Chu Xia walked out of the straw hut and did found some dragon-scale like grasses outside. She realized that these were the grasses that the young man in black had mentioned, and they were scales that the young man gave her. She was deeply moved. With tears, she dug many grass roots and went back.

初夏回去后,老中医用这种草药治疗怪病,疗效果然显著。初夏把她在龙潭的经历告诉了乡亲们,众乡亲也都非常感激那条小黑龙。为了表达他们的纪念之情,加上这种草根似蛟龙,叶似龙鳞,而且串根生长,生命力极强,于是乡亲们便把它叫作"穿山龙"。

After Chu Xia came back, her father used this grass root to make the herb soup, which was quite effective to the strange disease. Chu Xia told her story in Dragon Pond to her folks, and they were very grateful. The grasses Chu Xia had brought back had exuberant vitality and grew in strings. In order to memorize the black dragon, people called this grass with the dragon-like roots and the dragon scale-like leaves "dioscoreae nipponicae".

穿山龙味苦、性微寒。它的主要功效是祛风湿、活血通络、清肺化痰,多用于治疗风湿痹症和痰热咳喘。

The main medicinal virtues of dioscoreae nipponicae, which is bitter in taste and slightly cold in property, are expelling wind-dampness, activating blood circulation, removing obstruction in collaterals, clearing away heat from the lung and dissolving phlegm. It is often used for the treatment of rheumatic arthralgia and cough with asthma due to phlegm and heat in the lung.

第七章　党参

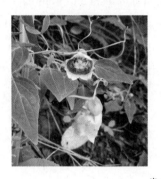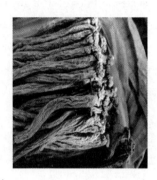

党参

Radix Codonopsis

古时候,有一个姓高的大财主,开了一家叫济世堂的中药铺。他在药铺里售卖很多假药和劣药,坑害一方百姓。

Chapter 7　Radix Codonopsis

In ancient times, there was a rich man named Gao, who ran a Chinese medicine pharmacy called Jishitang. He sold a lot of fake and inferior medicine in his pharmacy, bringing a lot of misfortune to the local people.

当地有一个叫张郎的家里很穷的年轻人,他的母亲吃了从这家药铺买的假药去世了。母亲死后,张郎和他父亲负债累累。不久,他的父亲也得了重病,张郎不得不来到济世堂赊购一些药。

There was a poor young man named Zhang Lang living in that area. His mother died after she took some fake medicine from this pharmacy. Zhang Lang and his father ran into debt after his mother's death. Before long, his father also became seriously ill. Zhang Lang had to come to Jishitang and bought some medicine on credit.

但是他父亲吃药后病情并没有改善,反而越发沉重了。原来,医生在处方上开的党参在抓药时被别的草药代替了。意识到自己不能依靠药铺里的药,张郎独自走进山里寻找党参。张郎背着背篓,拿着锄头,到山上四处寻找草药。

However, his father's condition was not improved but deteriorated after taking the medicine. It turned out that the radix codonopsis prescribed by the doctor was replaced by some other herbs in the pharmacy. Realizing that he couldn't rely on the medicine from the pharmacy, Zhang Lang went into the mountain to search for radix codonopsis by himself. With a basket on his back and a hoe in his hand, Zhang Lang went everywhere in the mountain to look for the herbs.

经过一天的攀爬,他感到筋疲力尽、饥饿难耐,黄昏时在一个山洞中晕倒了。他依稀感到自己似乎躺在花瓣覆盖的床上,床是如此柔软和舒适。在他面前站着一个美丽的年轻女孩,面目俊秀、身段苗条。

After a day's climbing, he felt so exhausted and hungry that he fainted in a cave at dusk. Vaguely he felt that he seemed to be lying on a petal-covered bed which was so soft and comfortable. In front of him stood a beautiful young girl with a pretty face and a slim figure.

女孩问他为什么来这里。听完他不幸的遭遇后,女孩说:"悬崖上两块大石头之间,有一棵很大的党参。你可以将它挖出并种植在园子里。摘一片叶子,煎煮一下给你父亲喝,他就会好起来的。"张郎突然醒了,原来是一场梦。

The girl asked him why he came here. After hearing his sad story, the girl said, "Between the two big rocks on the cliff there is a big radix codonopsis. You can dig it out and plant it in your garden. Pick a leaf and decoct it for your father to drink, and he will get better." Zhang Lang suddenly woke up. It turned out to be a dream.

这时候,天已经亮了。他爬上悬崖,发现了两块大石头。果然,在岩石中间有一棵很大的党参。他小心翼翼地把党参挖了出来。这棵党参很长,已经长成有胳膊和腿的人形模样,甚至还有眼睛和鼻子,酷似梦中的女孩。

At this time, it was dawning. He climbed up the cliff and found the two big rocks. Sure enough, there was a big radix codonopsis in the middle of the two rocks. He dug the herb out with tender care. This piece of radix codonopsis was very long and had already developed into human shape with arms and legs and even eyes and nose, resembling the girl in his dream very much.

他把党参和泥土放在一起,把藤和芽按顺序摆好,又把党参慢慢地放进背篓,一口气背回了家。他在园子里栽下党参,并为它搭了架子,然后摘下一片党参叶子煎煮后给父亲喝。几天后,父亲就康复了。

He put the radix codonopsis and the soil together, arranged the vines and sprouts in order, put the herb into his basket slowly and took it back home in one breath. After he planted the herb in his garden and set up a shelf for it he picked a leaf from the radix codonopsis and decocted it for his father to drink. Several days later, his father recovered.

从那时起,张郎每天都给党参浇水,还定期除草,把党参看得比什么都珍贵。有一天,梦中的美丽女孩从党参的藤架下面出现。于是他们结成了夫妻,幸福地生活在一起。

From then on, Zhang Lang watered the herb every day and weeded it regularly, valuing it very much. One day, the beautiful girl in his dream appeared from under the shelf of the radix codonopsis. They got married and lived happily together.

但是俗话说"世上没有不透风的墙"。那位姓高的财主很快就得知了这件事情。他逼迫张郎用园子里的党参和他美丽的妻子偿还债务。得知张郎不肯那样做，财主就来抢。但是园子里的党参和张郎的妻子一下子全消失了。

But as the saying goes, "There isn't a wall in the world which hasn't a crack." The rich man named Gao learned it very soon. He forced Zhang Lang to pay the debt with the herb in the garden and his beautiful wife. Seeing that Zhang Lang refused to do so, the rich man came to plunder them. But the herb in the garden and Zhang Lang's wife disappeared all at once.

财主恼羞成怒，就把张郎父子送到官府。官府的官员此前曾受过这个财主的贿赂，竟判了张郎"私种毒药，窝藏民女"的罪名，张郎披枷带镣，下入监牢。

The rich man was ashamed into anger. He then sent Zhang Lang and his father to the local government. The official, who had previously taken bribes from the rich man, convicted Zhang Lang of "growing poisonous herbs and hiding other's daughter privately". Zhang Lang was put into jail with shackles and chains.

回到山上后，这个化身党参的女孩发动了所有的草药仙子，如百合、柴胡、天麻、牡丹、桔梗和北沙参来施展法术。仙子们杀了县官和高财主，救出了张郎。夫妻双双回到了山上。后来张郎也化身为一种叫作"黄花"的药材。

After the girl who was the embodiment of radix codonopsis returned to the mountain, she gathered all the fairies of medical herbs such as lily bulb, bupleurum, gastrodia, peony, platycodon root and glehnia to make a magic. The fairies killed the local official and the rich man. Zhang Lang was saved and went to the mountain together with his wife. Later, Zhang Lang turned into another medical herb called "*huanghua*".

党参性平、味甘,补中益气。党参之名,最早的记载见于清代吴仪洛所撰《本草从新》:"参须上党者佳。今真党参久已难得,肆中所卖党参,种类甚多,皆不堪用。唯防风党参,性味和平足贵,根有狮子盘头者真,硬纹者伪也。"

Known for its health-giving qualities, radix codonopsis is mild-natured, sweet, and is said to tonify spleen-stomach and replenish *qi* (or stamina). The book *New Compilation of Materia Medica* by Wu Yiluo in the Qing Dynasty left the earliest record about radix codonopsis, "Radix codonopsis comes into flourishing term in Shangdang, China's Shanxi Province. A real one is hard to come by nowadays. The markets are flooded with various kinds of so-called radix codonopsis which are suitable for decorative purpose but unsuitable for utility. Among these TCM ingredients, only *fangfeng* and radix codonopsis are mild in taste and nature which make their existing properties all the more valuable. A real radix codonopsis is commonly depicted in its vivid animal form, with a lion-like tuberculate stem traces-covered head at the root, while a fake one only has hard lines in its root area."

第八章 地骨皮

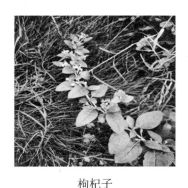

枸杞子
Fructus Lycii

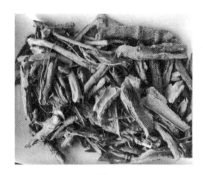

地骨皮
Cortex Lycii

地骨皮又名"枸杞根皮",为什么会把枸杞根皮叫作"地骨皮"呢?这其中还有一段传说。

Chapter 8 Cortex Lycii

Cortex lycii is also known as the root skin of Chinese wolfberry, but why? There is a legend about it.

相传有一天,大清的慈禧太后感觉胸闷,视物模糊,御医们全都束手无策。可巧这时有位姓钱的将军对御医们说起了一件事。他的母亲以前也曾患过类似的病,后来被一位妙手回春的民间医生治好了。这位医生挖来枸杞根,洗净后剥下枸杞根皮,叮嘱钱将军用其煎汤给母亲服用,后来钱将军的母亲就病愈了。御医们听到这些,就举荐钱将军献药方。

According to legend, one day, Empress Dowager Ci Xi of the Qing Dynasty felt chest tightness and a blurred vision. All the imperial physicians failed to cure the disease. It so happened that General Qian mentioned to the imperial physicians that his mother used to suffer from similar problem and was cured by a famous practitioner of folk medicine who could bring the dying back to life. The doctor first dug out the root of cortex lycii, peeled off the root skin of Chinese wolfberry after washing it clean, and then decocted them with water. General Qian's mother drank the decoction and recovered soon. On hearing this, these imperial physicians recommended the general and his prescription to Empress Dowager Ci Xi.

慈禧太后立即下诏，命钱将军返乡取药。钱将军从家乡带回一大包枸杞根皮，亲自在太医院煎好汤药，送至宫中，服侍慈禧太后用药。几天后，慈禧太后果然觉得眼明心亮，精神渐涨，便问钱将军用了何种良方妙药。

Empress Dowager Ci Xi immediately ordered the general to go back to his hometown to fetch the herbs. The general brought back a large parcel of root skin of Chinese wolfberry from his hometown, decocted by himself in the Imperial Academy of Medicine and sent the decoction to the Empress Dowager Ci Xi. Several days later, having drunk this herb, Empress Dowager Ci Xi gradually was sharp-eyed and clear-headed, and had much better mental outlook. So she asked the general about the name of this magic herb.

钱将军思忖，枸杞的"枸"和"狗"同音，如实禀报，太后定会不悦，琢磨了半天，便择了个吉祥的名称"地骨皮"。慈禧老佛爷不由得拊掌赞叹说："好哇！哀家食用地骨之皮，可与天地长寿！"从那以后，枸杞根就被称为地骨皮了。

The general pondered that one sound of the Chinese wolfberry sounded like "*gou*" (dog). If he told the truth to the Empress Dowager Ci Xi, the offending word would definitely give rise to displeasure. Turning over the name in his mind for quite a while, finally he gave it a luckier name "*digupi*". The Empress Dowager Ci Xi couldn't help clapping her hands and gasped in admiration, "That's great! I have taken the *digupi*, and could live as long as the heaven and the earth." Since then, the root skin of Chinese wolfberry came to be known as *digupi* (cortex lycii).

地骨皮药性甘、寒,主要功效为凉血退蒸、清肺降火。

Cortex lycii has a cold nature and sweet flavor, and has long been thought to have benefits ranging from cooling blood, relieving bone-steaming, clearing away the lung-heat to removing pathogenic fire.

第九章　地龙

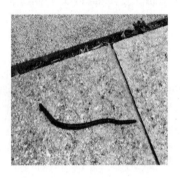 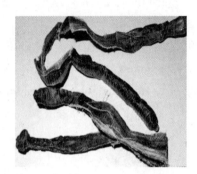

地龙
Pheretima

相传宋太祖赵匡胤登基不久，就患了"蛇缠腰"，他的哮喘病也一并复发。宫里的太医们殚精竭虑也无回春之术。赵匡胤一怒之下，把所有治病的太医抓进了大牢。

Chapter 9　Pheretima

Legend had it that soon after Zhao Kuangyin, the founding emperor of the Song Dynasty ascended the throng, he suffered from herpes zoster, along with the recurrence of the old disease asthma. All the imperial physicians racked their brains but his illness took no favourable turn. The emperor got so furious that he put all of them into prison.

一天，一位太医突然想起洛阳有个擅长治疗皮肤病的药铺掌柜，医术精妙，人送绰号"活洞宾"，太医就把他推荐给了赵匡胤。"活洞宾"很快奉旨来到宫中，仔细查看赵匡胤的病情，只见他身上环腰布满了一串串豆粒大的水疱。

One day, it suddenly occurred to one imperial physician that there was a herbal medicine shopkeeper in Luoyang City, who was proficient in treating the skin problems and thus got a nickname of "living Dongbin" (a legendary figure in China). The imperial physician then recommended him to the emperor. Soon the "living Dongbin" came on imperial orders. A closer look at it revealed that many blisters as big as the peas were around the emperor's waist.

赵匡胤威严地问道："朕的病情如何？""活洞宾"回道："皇上不必担忧，有药可治，用上几次便可痊愈。"赵匡胤冷笑道："太医们都无良策，你怎敢说此大话？""活洞宾"道："倘若治不好皇上的病，小民情愿杀头；若治好了，小民有一事相求，就是放了那些被监禁的太医们。"太祖应允。

The emperor asked imperially how sick he might be. The "living Dongbin" responded, "You need not worry. I have the cure. You will be all right after using it several times." The emperor sneered, "All the imperial physicians failed to give treatment. How dare you say that?" The "living Dongbin" replied, "If I fail to give a cure, you may cut off my head as a punishment. But if I succeed, I just beg you one thing. I beg you to free all these imperial physicians in the prison." The emperor gave a nod of assent.

于是，"活洞宾"来到大殿一角，打开药罐，取出几条蚯蚓放在两个盘子里，涂抹上蜂蜜。不一会儿，蚯蚓就化成了液体。"活洞宾"用棉花蘸上这些液体，涂抹在太祖的患处，太祖很快就感到浑身清凉舒适。"活洞宾"又奉上另一瓶药汁请太祖服下，太祖诧异："这是何药？既可外用，又能内服？"

The "living Dongbin" then came to one corner of the palace, open the traditional decoction gallipot and took several earthworms out from it. He put the earthworms in a plate and smeared honey on them. After a while, the earthworms dissolved into liquid. The "living Dongbin" wiped the liquid on the emperor's affected part, and the emperor soon felt cool and comfortable. The "living Dongbin" then served the other plate of the liquid to the emperor, suggesting him to drink up. The emperor got very surprised, "What's this? Can it be used both internally and externally?"

"活洞宾"怕告知真情太祖不肯服药,便顺势言道:"皇上乃真龙天子,民间俗药怎能奏效？此药名'地龙',龙补龙方有神效。"太祖听了十分高兴,端起药一饮而尽。几天后,太祖的病便痊愈了。从此,"地龙"的大名就广为流传了。

The "living Dongbin" didn't tell the emperor the truth for fear that the emperor would not take the medicine. He answered, "You are the true dragon and son of heaven, the normal medicine on earth was unfit for you. This medicine is "*dilong*" (dragon on earth), which fits the real dragon like you." On hearing these words, the emperor got very pleased and drank it off. Several days later, the emperor recovered. Since then, the name of "*dilong*" (dragon on earth) was widely spread.

地龙性咸、味寒,能清热定惊、通络、平喘、利尿。

Being salty and cold, pheretima (earthworm) allows a legion of medical uses, covering clearing heat and tranquilizing, removing obstructions in collaterals, relieving asthma and promoting urination.

第十章　丁公藤

　　清朝黄小坪撰写的《百孝图记·药医》一书记载了"解叔谦藤酒疗亲"的故事。南北朝时期，山西雁门关附近住着一个叫解叔谦的人，解叔谦素来孝顺，他侍奉久病不愈的母亲，备受乡邻称赞。在夜深人静的时候，他在院子里虔诚地对天祈祷。恍惚间他听到空中有人对他说："你母亲的病没有什么可担忧的，只要用丁公藤制酒饮下，便可痊愈。"

Chapter 10　Caulis Erycibes

丁公藤
Caulis Erycibes

　　As recorded in the book *One Hundred Stories about Filial Behavior* compiled by Huang Xiaoping in the Qing Dynasty, during the Southern and Northern Dynasties (420 A.D.-589 A.D.), there lived a man named Xie Shuqian near Yanmen Pass in Shanxi Province. He was showered with praise from his neighbors due to his filial piety to his mother who suffered from a long period of uncured disease. At night when all was still, he prayed to the heaven piously in the yard for his mother's illness. Deep in a trance, he heard a voice in the air, "You have nothing to worry about, and your mother will be fine as long as she drinks the wine made by caulis erycibes."

　　解叔谦大吃一惊，但见空中什么也没有，只有余音萦绕在耳边。第二天，他就遍访懂得药理的人，向他们询问丁公藤，大家都茫然不解。接着他又查遍各种方书和草药，也没有这种药名。叔谦甚为焦灼，神明既然有此明示，就绝不可能没有丁公藤。于是解叔谦就外出访问，但仍然没有人知道，他心里甚为懊丧，发誓不找到丁公藤决不罢休。

Xie Shuqian's immediate reaction was one of shock. He found nothing in the sky, and only the ethereal voices lingered around his ears. The next day, he made contact with everyone with an idea for pharmacology to enquire about caulis erycibes, but they were all quite at a loss. He then combed through all kinds of medical formularies and herbs, but still found no traces of it. He was deeply worried. Since the gods gave clear clues, there's definitely one herb named caulis erycibes. Thus he went out to hear from anyone who knew this herb, but they all disclaimed any knowledge of caulis erycibes. Though he felt frustrated at the lack of progress, he swore he would never give up until he reached his goal.

待他到了宜都（今属湖北），路过一座山时，忽然看见一个老汉正在用斧头砍伐树木，树的形状不同寻常。解叔谦心里一动，急忙上前问道："这是什么树？您砍伐它作何用途？"老汉答道："这种树的名字知道的人很少。您既然问我，我就欣然奉告。这就是丁公藤，治疗风湿病有特效。用它泡酒，让病人喝下，灵验无比。"老汉当即赠给他几段丁公藤，并说明了泡酒的方法。

When he arrived at Yidu (now part of Hubei) and was passing through a mountain, suddenly his eyes caught sight of an old man chopping an unusual tree with an axe. Seized by a sudden inspiration, he approached and asked hurriedly, "What is it? What do you usually use the tree for?" "Few know the tree's name." the old man replied. "Now that you asked me, I am pleased to inform you that this is caulis erycibes which deals with rheumatism with special effects. This medicine is highly efficacious if it is soaked in wine for a drink." The old man presented him with several segments of caulis erycibes right away and explained the method of steeping in wine.

解叔谦拜谢老汉，收下了丁公藤，倏忽间老汉消失得无影无踪。解叔谦知道这是神明的指示，就携带丁公藤返回家中，按照老汉说的方法炮制药酒，让母亲饮用，母亲的风湿病果然奇迹般地痊愈了。

Xie Shuqian expressed his thanks to the old man and accepted the caulis erycibes. Just seconds later, the old man disappeared without any trace. Xie Shuqian knew it was a divine direction, so he brought the caulis erycibes home and prepared the medicated wine according to the old man's instructions. Sure enough, his mother made a miraculous recovery after the wine had been served to her.

丁公藤味辛、性温，有微毒，能祛风湿、消肿止痛，主要应用于风湿痹痛、半身不遂和跌打损伤。

Caulis erycibes is characterized by warm nature, pungent flavors and slight toxicity, and has medicinal virtues of expelling rheumatism, relieving swelling and alleviating pain. Clinically, it has been applied to rheumatic arthralgia, hemiplegia and traumatic injury.

第十一章 杜鹃花

关于杜鹃花的由来,有一段传说。闽东山区杜家村住着一户穷苦人家,家中有母亲和两个儿子。大儿子30多岁还没娶媳妇,村里人都叫他杜一。二儿子杜二刚过16岁。兄弟俩以贩卖私盐为生,奉养老母。杜一正值壮年,力气大,一次可挑盐140千克,而杜二力气单薄,一担不过40千克,一家人省吃俭用地过日子,勉强糊口。

Chapter 11 Rhododendron

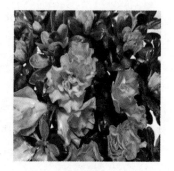

杜鹃花
Rhododendron

When it comes to rhododendron, there is a legend about it. In the mountain area of the eastern Fujian Province, there lived a poor family with a mother and two sons in Dujia Village. The elder son, known as Du Yi, was still unmarried in his thirties. The younger brother, Du Er, had recently turned 16. The brothers made a living by selling the illegal salt to support their mother. At the prime working age, Du Yi could carry 140kg salt each time because of his great strength. While Du Er had weak strength and could carry no more than 40kg salt each time. The family led their lives, pinching and scraping, living from hand to mouth.

有一天,杜一路过大街歇脚的时候,由于担子太重,盐担滑落,压死了一个小孩。杜一被官府抓去,关在牢里,判了斩刑。杜二一个人卖盐,养活老母,日子过得十分艰难。有一次,杜一对前来探监的弟弟说:"再过7天,我就要被带去刑场了。"兄弟俩抱头痛哭。弟弟说:"让我替你死吧。我力气小,挣的钱难以养活母亲,最终我们都会饿死。我死便死一个,你死便死三个。"说完弟弟把哥哥推出门外,自己进了牢房。

  One day, Du Yi stopped on the way for a rest in a street. His salt load was so heavy that it fell down and ran over a child. Therefore, Du Yi was caught by the feudal officials, put into prison and sentenced to death. Du Er had a harsh time for he could not sell enough salt to care for their old mother. Once Du Yi said to his younger brother who came to see him, "In seven days, I will be taken to the execution ground." The two brothers cried on each other's shoulders. Du Er said, "Let me replace you to die. I have weak strength and cannot earn enough money to look after our mother. We will starve to death in the end. If I die, you and mum could survive. But if you die, all of us could not live any longer." With these words, the younger brother pushed the elder brother out of the cell and stepped into prison.

  过了一周,杜二做了替死鬼。可是杜一胆小怕事,出狱后并没有回家侍奉老母,而是躲起来了。杜二的灵魂化作杜鹃鸟,到处喊叫:"哥哥回来!哥哥回来!"一边叫,一边口中滴着鲜血,鲜血所洒之处,长出了杜鹃花。从那以后,每年春天漫山遍野都会开出一片红色的杜鹃花,人们都说,这是杜二的一片丹心与孝心。

  Seven days later, Du Er was made a scapegoat. But Du Yi was so timid and overcautious that he hid somewhere instead of returning home to attend to his mother. The soul of Du Er turned into a cuckoo, crying out everywhere with blood dripping from its mouth, "Brother, come back! Brother, come back!" The blood sprinkled and the rhododendron grew. Since then, red rhododendron blossomed all over the mountain every spring, which was known as Du Er's loyal heart and filial piety.

  就在杜二的灵魂到处找哥哥的时候,村里人发现,距杜家村数十里的大山后面,经常有一群山羊仰天喊叫:"妈妈!妈妈!"好奇的村民进山查看,发现离羊群不远处有一具腐尸,从衣服来看,这就是杜一,他的尸体旁长出了一株有毒的杜鹃。

While the soul of Du Er was looking for his brother, behind a huge mountain, miles away from Dujia Village, the villagers found that a herd of goats frequently threw back their heads and cried, "Mom! Mom!" The curious villagers went into the mountain and found a cankered corpse a short distance away from the goats. Judging from the clothes, it was Du Yi. Beside the corpse a toxic rhododendron sprouted out.

后来,杜鹃花就被用作一味可以止咳、平喘、祛痰的中药。

Later, rhododendron is used as a kind of Chinese herb with efficacies of relieving cough, asthma and eliminating phlegm.

第十二章 独一味

相传三国时期,有一天,一个姓王的士兵在西康省瞻化县(今四川省甘孜藏族自治州的新龙县)的野外放军马,被一伙拦路抢劫的强盗一箭射中了大腿。这姓王的士兵四下环顾,发现一个人都没有,他伤势很重,又无力喊叫,料得性命难保,他只能眼望着辽阔的草原,坐以待毙。

Chapter 12　Lamiophlomis Rotata

According to legend, during Three Kingdoms Period, one day, a soldier surnamed Wang was assaulted by a gang of robbers and was shot by an arrow in his right thigh when he was herding army horses in the wild in Zhanhua County of Xikang Province (now Xinlong County of Ganzi Tibetan Autonomous Prefecture, southwest China's Sichuan Province). Looking around, he found nobody anywhere. He wanted to shout loudly, but was badly wounded and too weak to call for help. He felt that he would come to the end of life and could do nothing but stare at the vast grassland, waiting for death.

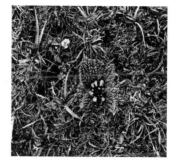

独一味

Lamiophlomis Rotata

过了一会儿,草原上的一股冷风把士兵吹醒。这时他伤口感染,疼痛难耐,便萌生了自行了断的念头。他按住伤口,忍着剧烈的疼痛,艰难地爬向军营。他无意中发现身边有一种小草长得十分惹人喜爱,便顺手连根拔起一棵,抖落泥土,放入嘴中咀嚼。虽然这草的味道有点苦,但对于他来说,可以让自己不那么痛苦。士兵身上的伤口流血不止,他又将小草嚼碎,敷在伤口处。

A moment later, the cold wind woke him. Now the wound from an arrow had become infected and the unbearable pain provoked suicidal thoughts. He pressed the wound, endured the severe pain and crawled hardly to the barracks. Accidentally, he found an appealing grass at his side and pulled up one with root. Shaking the mud off, he put it into mouth and chewed it. Though it was bitter, it might be able to ease his pain for him. Uncontrolled bleeding from his wound stirred him to chew the grass and coat it on the wound.

过了一会儿，士兵感觉疼痛减轻了许多，伤口处渐渐消肿，他终于在深夜爬回了营地。不可思议的是，过了几天他的伤口竟然痊愈了。

After a while, the wound was giving him much less pain and little by little the swelling was gone. He eventually crawled back to the barracks in the dead of night. It was incredible that the wound was healed unexpectedly a few days later.

官兵们见这个士兵的箭伤好得如此之快，都很好奇，就追问起药物的来龙去脉。士兵从衣服口袋里拿出小草说："就是这单独一味草药医治好了我的箭伤。"众人都惊奇地喊出："是独一味呀！"从那时起，"独一味"的大名很快就流传开了。

The officers and soldiers were all curious about his quick recovery and probed into the ins and outs of the matter. The soldier took out the grass from his pocket and said, "This particular single herb saved me." The officers and soldiers let out a cry of surprise, "It's really *duyiwei* (the only and unique one)!" From that moment on, the name of *duyiwei* (lamiophlomis rotata) soon spread across the nation.

独一味味苦、性微寒，归肝经，具有活血止血、祛风止痛之功效，适用于跌打损伤、外伤出血、风湿痹痛和黄水病。但独一味是一种有毒植物，所以使用时要遵照医嘱，以免中毒伤身。

Lamiophlomis rotata is bitter in taste, a little cold in nature and attributive to liver. The pooled clinically efficacy information has shown that it is very efficient at invigorating the circulation of blood, arresting hemorrhage, dispersing pathogenic wind and alleviating pains. It has long been thought to go for traumatic injury, bleeding due to trauma, rheumatic arthralgia together with diseases caused by dampness and damp-heat. This herb is known to possess toxicity, thus it is advisable to act on the doctor's advice to avoid poisoning.

第十三章　杜仲

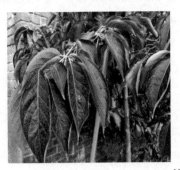 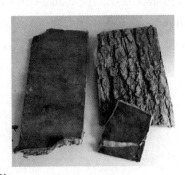

杜仲
Eucommia Ulmoides

很久以前，洞庭湖畔的货物主要靠木船来运输，岸上光着脚拉纤的纤夫们由于经年累月低头弯腰拉纤，积劳成疾，多半会腰膝疼痛。看到大伙儿的这种状况，有一名叫杜仲的年轻纤夫心急如焚，他一心想寻得一味草药来消除大家的病痛。

Chapter 13　Eucommia Ulmoides

Long long ago, the goods by Dongting Lake were transported mainly by wooden boats. Most of the barefooted boat trackers on the shore suffered severe pains in waist and knees for they bent to tow boats with their heads down year in year out. On seeing this, a young boat tracker named Du Zhong was burning with anxiety. His only thought was to find the medicine to eliminate the pains.

告别了家人，杜仲背着行囊上山采药。有一天，他在山上遇到了一位鹤发童颜的老翁，于是上前拜见，可老翁头也不回地走了。杜仲离家已一月有余，所带的口粮也已经吃光，可至今还未找到草药，心下不免焦急。于是，他又快步追上前去拜求老翁，倾诉了纤夫们的疾苦。老翁深为感动，从药篓中取出一块树皮递给杜仲，指着对面巍峨的高山再三叮嘱："这树皮能治腰膝疼痛，但此山崎岖险峻，一定要小心啊！"杜仲连声道谢，拜别了老翁，直奔那崇山峻岭而去。

Carrying packs, Du Zhong bade farewell to his family and went into the hills to gather herbs. One day, he met an old herb collector with white hair and ruddy complexion on the mountain. He then marched forward to pay respects, but the old man left without looking back. Du Zhong had been away from home for more than a month and the food prepared was almost eaten up. His heart was torn with anxiety for he still did not have any clue of the herb yet. He then walked quickly and caught the old man, pouring out the sufferings of the boat trackers. Being deeply moved, the old man brought out a piece of bark from his medicine basket and gave it to Du Zhong. Pointing at the towering mountain in the opposite, the old man told him once again, "This bark can possibly cure the pain, but the mountain is precipitous and dangerous, be careful!" Du Zhong expressed his thanks and said goodbye to him. Then he went straight to the high mountains and lofty hills.

行至半路，杜仲又偶遇一位老樵夫。老樵夫听说他要上山顶采药，急忙劝阻："年轻人，想必你是不知道凶险啊，此山巅鸟儿也插翅难飞，猿猴也难为攀爬，此去凶多吉少啊。"

On halfway, Du Zhong encountered an old woodcutter. When he heard that Du Zhong intended to collect herbs at the peak of the mountain, the old woodcutter dissuaded him from doing that hurriedly, "Young man, presumably you have a dim idea of the dangerous situation. This mountain peak is too high for birds to fly over and too tough for monkeys to climb up. Everything points to a disaster."

杜仲决意要为纤夫们解除病痛,于是毫不犹豫地往上攀爬。爬至半山腰,他腹中饥饿,头晕眼花,突然滚落山崖,所幸身子悬挂在一棵大树上。过了一会儿,他苏醒了过来,发现身边正是自己要找的那种树,于是就强撑着拼命采集树皮,但因为体力不支,最后他精疲力竭,被山水冲入了洞庭湖。

Without any hesitation, Du Zhong began to struggle up the mountain for he made up his mind to relieve sufferings of the boat trackers. Halfway up the mountain he was so hungry that he had a dizzy head and blurred eyes. Suddenly he toppled over the cliff but fortunately was hung by a big tree. After a while, he came to life and found the tree he sought was just beside him. So he desperately strived to collect the bark. Finally he was so tired physically and exhausted that he was rushed into Dongting Lake by the water from the mountain.

洞庭湖畔的纤夫们听闻这一噩耗,悲痛不已,立刻开始寻找杜仲的下落。当他们最终找到他的尸体时,发现他还紧紧地抱着一捆新采集的树皮。纤夫们噙着泪水吃完了他采集的树皮,神奇的事情发生了,他们的腰膝疼痛果真好了。为了纪念杜仲,纤夫们就将此树皮命名为"杜仲"。

On hearing the sad news, the boat trackers by Dongting Lake were grieving over his death and started to search him immediately. When they finally found Du Zhong's body, they found that he held a bundle of newly-collected barks tightly. Boat trackers ate up all these barks with tears. Then the magical thing happened, their pains in waist and knees were cured as expected. In memory of Du Zhong, the bark was named after him by the boat trackers.

杜仲味甘、性温,归肝肾,能补肝肾、强筋骨,多用于肾虚及各种腰痛。

Eucommia ulmoides is featured by sweet flavor and warm nature, and ascribes to liver and kidney. The power of eucommia ulmoides lies in nourishing liver and kidney, and strengthening tendons and bones. Clinically, most of its interventions for patients are with deficiency of kidney and various lumbagos.

第十四章 阿胶

阿胶

Ejiao

相传唐朝时期,阿城镇上住着一对靠贩驴为生的恩爱夫妻,男的叫阿铭,女的叫阿桥。

Chapter 14 *Ejiao*

Local legend had it that there lived a loving couple in the A'cheng Town in the Tang Dynasty who made a living by peddling donkeys. The husband's name was Ming and the wife's name was Qiao.

结婚两年后,阿桥怀孕了。但是阿桥分娩后因气血损耗,身体变得很虚弱,整日卧病在床,吃了很多补气血的药,丝毫不见好转。阿铭听说驴肉滋补身体,便想让阿桥尝试一下,也许这会帮助她恢复身体。

After two years of marriage, Qiao got pregnant. After giving birth, however, she became very weak due to loss of *qi* and blood. Therefore, she was confined to bed all day long. She took a lot of medicine to invigorate *qi* and enrich blood, but nothing worked. Ming heard that the meat of donkey served as a good recipe for nourishing the body, so he wanted Qiao to have a try, maybe it would assist with her recovery.

于是,阿铭就让伙计宰了一头小毛驴,把肉放在锅里煮。谁知煮肉的伙计闻到香味,引出了馋虫,肉一煮熟便从锅里捞出来吃。其他伙计闻到香味,也围过来吃,这个尝一口,那个尝一口,不一会儿一锅驴肉全被吃光了。

So Ming asked one of his assistants to slaughter a donkey and boil the meat in a pot. Unexpectedly, the assistant was so gluttonous that he couldn't resist the temptation to eat the meat as soon as it was done. The other assistants gathered around and competed to eat when they smelled the aroma. In a moment the assistants snarfed up all the meat.

煮肉的伙计看这情形着了慌,女主人吃什么呢?迫于无奈,他只好把剩下的驴皮切碎放进锅里熬。熬了半天才把驴皮熬化了。伙计把熬制的浓浓的驴皮汤从锅里舀出来倒进盆里,驴皮汤冷却后竟然凝固成黏糊糊的胶块。伙计尝了一口,觉得还算可口,于是就把这驴皮胶端给阿桥吃。

At this moment the assistant who boiled the meat began to worry. What would the hostess eat? He had no choice but to cut the skin of the donkey into small pieces and boiled them again. It took him nearly half a day to make it ready. The assistant scooped the thick donkey skin soup and poured it into the pot. As it cooled, it was solidified into a sticky gel. The assistant took a sip of it and found it palatable. So he sent it to Qiao.

阿桥平时没有吃过驴肉,尝了一口,觉得食欲大增,竟然很快就把一盆驴皮胶全吃光了。几天后,奇迹出现了,她面色红润、气血充沛,整个人都有了精神。

Qiao had never eaten donkey meat before. She took a bite and found it appetite-boosting. She soon ate up the whole basin of donkey-skin soup. Several days later, there came a miracle. Qiao had a ruddy complexion and sufficient *qi* and blood. She felt that she was full of energy.

一年后，那位伙计的妻子也分娩了。由于家里穷，他的妻子怀孕期间营养不良，分娩后身体十分虚弱。伙计请了郎中开了许多补药，但都无济于事。伙计忽然想起阿桥吃驴皮胶那档事儿来。于是，便将当时熬驴皮的事情向阿铭夫妇和盘托出，并且希望能向他们夫妻借头毛驴。阿桥心肠软，见他十分焦急就动了恻隐之心，答应了伙计的请求。

A year later, the assistant's wife also gave birth to a baby. The mere fact of being poor gave rise to her malnutrition during the pregnancy which made her very weak after the delivery. The assistant sought a doctor for a prescription of a lot of tonics, but the medicine didn't work. Suddenly an idea flashed into his mind that his wife could also try the donkey-skin soup just like Qiao. The whole story of boiling the donkey skin soup then came pouring out to Ming and Qiao, and the assistant hoped they would look kindly on his request of borrowing a donkey from them. Qiao's soft heart was touched by his anxiousness, so she agreed to his request.

伙计牵回毛驴，把驴皮熬成胶块给妻子吃。果然不出几日，妻子便大有起色。从此以后，驴皮胶是产妇的大补良药就在百姓们中间传开了。阿铭夫妇开始经营驴皮胶生意。有些人见熬驴皮胶有利可图，也争相仿效。可奇怪的是，只有阿城当地熬出的驴皮胶才有疗效，这就引起了纠纷。官司打到县里，县太爷带着郎中来到阿城一探虚实。他们发现阿城镇水井里的水与其他地方的大不相同。

The assistant led a donkey back home, boiled the donkey's skin to gel and gave it to his wife to eat. Sure enough, several days later his wife felt much better. From then on, it became widely known that the donkey skin served as good medicine for lying-in women due to its nourishing effect. Ming and Qiao began to run a business of donkey-hide gelatin. It was so profitable that many people followed. Strangely enough, only the gel produced in A'cheng was effective. Then disputes arose and the official of the county came to find out the truth with a doctor. After investigation, they found that the water in the well of A'cheng Town was quite different from that in other places.

县太爷又惊又喜,才知道驴胶熬制有赖于当地得天独厚的井水。于是他下令今后只有阿城镇才能熬胶。县令还将驴皮胶进贡给当朝皇上李世民。李世民把驴皮胶赏赐给年迈体弱的大臣,大臣们吃了阿胶后发现其果然是上等的补品。李世民差大将尉迟恭来到阿城,召集匠人将阿城的水井修葺一新,并在井上加盖了一座亭子,亭子里竖立石碑。迄今为止,碑文上刻的"唐朝钦差大臣尉迟恭至此重修阿井"字样还依稀可见。

The official was both surprised and delighted on hearing this. He then came to know that the making of donkey-skin gel relied upon the advantaged water in the local well. He not only ordered that only the people in A'cheng Town had the rights to make the gel, but also paid the gel as a tribute to the Emperor Li Shimin. The emperor gave it as a reward to the ministers who were suffering from age and infirmity. It turned out to be first-class tonic. An imperial edict then brought general Yuchi Gong to A'cheng Town and every available craftsman was called to rebuild the well in the town. A pavilion rose up from the well, in which a stone tablet was erected. Up till now, the tablet inscription "Imperial Envoy Yuchi Gong of the Tang Dynasty Rebuilt the Well" is just discernible.

阿胶作为一味大众耳熟能详的滋补药材,原产地为山东省阿县,现今阿胶均以山东东阿驴皮阿胶为上品。阿胶最初盛行于宫廷,后来才在民间普及。其应用的记载最早可追溯到《神农本草经》。明朝李时珍所撰《本草纲目》也有关于其功效的论述,该书将驴皮阿胶列为"圣药"。

As a familiar refrain, *ejiao*, a gelatin made of donkey hides, is a kind of tonifying medicinal materials. Nowadays Shandong province-based Dong'e *ejiao*, the country's top maker of hallmarked TCM products, has been scheduled as a top grade. *Ejiao* first prevailed in the imperial family and later gained popularity among the general public. The earliest record of it could be traced back to the classic *Shennong's Classic of Materia Medica*. Donkey-hide gelatin was dubbed a "Holy Medicine" long ago by Li Shizhen, the author of *Compendium of Materia Medica* in the Ming Dynasty which gave an exposition of the efficacies of *ejiao*.

第十五章　茯苓

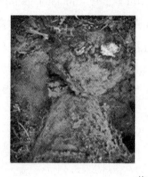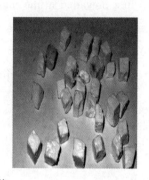

茯苓

Poria Cocos

传说从前有个员外,膝下育有一女,取名苓儿。员外家还雇了一个青壮年男子管理家务,叫作茯儿。茯儿老实勤快,员外家的小姐暗暗地爱上了他。不料员外知道后,雷霆大怒。他嫌贫爱富,不愿把女儿嫁给茯儿。他准备把茯儿赶走,把自己的女儿关起来,并且要将她许配给一个富家公子。二人得知此事后,便一起从家里逃了出来,住进了一个偏僻的小村庄。

Chapter 15　Poria Cocos

According to Chinese legends, in the past, there was a ministry councilor who had a daughter named Ling. The ministry councilor hired a strong young man named Fu to help him keep house. Ling fell in love with this diligent and honest young man, only to find her father flew into a rage after knowing all this. Despising the poor and currying favour with the rich, he could not assent their marriage. Therefore, he decided to drive him away and lock his daughter up in the room with the intention of marrying her to a rich man. On hearing this, Ling and Fu secretly fled away from home and settled down in a remote small village.

苓儿离开家之后得了风湿病,卧床不起,茯儿不眠不休,日夜照顾她,他与妻子同甘共苦,对她坚贞不渝。
After leaving home, Ling was bedridden with rheumatic disease. Fu took after her all day and all night tirelessly. He stuck faithfully to his wife through thick and thin.

有一天,茯儿进山为苓儿采药,忽见前面有只雪白的野兔正在回头看他,他一箭射中野兔,野兔却带伤跑掉了,茯儿紧追不舍,追到了一片松林处,野兔忽然不见了。他四处寻找,最后发现在一棵松树旁边,一个棕黑色的球形的东西上面插着他的那支箭。茯儿拔起箭仔细查看,他发现这个球体表皮裂口处,白似番薯。他把这个东西带回家,煮熟了给苓儿吃。
One day, Fu went into the mountain to collect herbs for Ling. A white rabbit which kept looking back at him was suddenly seen. He shot an arrow at the rabbit, but the rabbit ran away with injuries. He followed closely behind it, and found the rabbit disappeared in a forest with many pine trees. He looked around for any signs of it, and eventually found his arrow in a brownish black ball-shaped stuff near a pine tree. He pulled out the arrow and examined it carefully. There were many cracks outside and it was as white as sweet potato inside. He took it home and cooked it for Ling.

第二天,苓儿就觉得浑身上下舒服多了,茯儿喜不自胜,便经常挖这些东西给苓儿吃,苓儿的风湿病逐渐痊愈了。消息传开了,大家都知道了这药的神效。由于它是茯儿和苓儿最先发现的,人们就把它叫作"茯苓"。

The next day, Ling felt much better all over. Overwhelmed with joy, Fu was habitually engaged in digging such stuff for his wife. Gradually Ling recovered. This news soon got around. Now everyone knew the magical effect of this herb. It was called *"fuling"* (poria cocos) because it was first discovered by Fu and Ling.

茯苓始载于目前我国发现最早的医学方书《五十二病方》,以"服零"呈现。《神农本草经》将其归于上品,记为"伏苓"。茯苓味甘、性平,具有利水渗湿、健脾安神等功效。因其功效广泛,四季均可服用,古人称其为"四时神药"。

The earliest discovered traces of poria cocos was in the oldest extant medical formulary found in China, *Recipes for 52 Kinds of Disorders*, in which poria cocos took on the form of "服零". *Shennong's Classic of Materia Medica* ascribed poria cocos to top grade of the line, and made it appear to be the form of "伏苓". Being sweet and mild-natured, poria cocos has a range of efficacies that go from facilitating diuresis, draining dampness, invigorating spleen to relieving uneasiness of mind, etc. Poria cocos, described by the ancients as a "Four-Season Miracle Cure", is universally applicable in all seasons.

第十六章　枸杞子

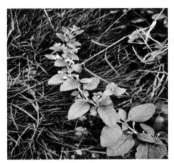 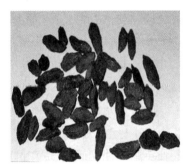

枸杞子
Fructus Lycii

盛唐时期,丝绸之路是东西方贸易和文化交流汇融之道。有一天,一队西域商人经由丝绸之路来到长安,为首的是个"中国通"。傍晚在客栈住宿,见一十五六岁的少女斥责鞭打一位八九十岁的老翁。这位"中国通"义愤填膺,便上前责问道:"你为何这般责打老人?"

Chapter 16 Fructus Lycii

During the flourishing period of the Tang Dynasty, the ancient Silk Road served as a way for East and West trade, cultural exchanges and integration. One day, a team of merchants from the Western Regions traveled the Silk Road to Chang'an. At dusk the team which was headed by an "old China hand" stayed at an inn. The "old China hand" was filled with indignation when he saw a girl at the age of 15 or 16 was scolding and lashing an old man in his eighties or nineties. He went forward and asked reprovingly, "Why do you scold and beat the old man?"

那少女言道:"我责罚自己的曾孙,与你有什么相干?"这位"中国通"大吃一惊。原来,这女子竟然已经372岁,老翁也已90多岁,他被责打是因为不肯服用草药,弄得未老先衰、两鬓斑白、两眼昏花。

The girl responded, "I punish my great-grandson. It's none of your business!" The "old China hand" gasped with surprise at her words. The girl turned out to be 372 years old, and the old man was over 90. He was scolded and beaten for his unwillingness of taking herbal medicine, which led to his premature aging, grey hair and blurred vision.

听闻此言,这位"中国通"越发惊讶好奇,忙作揖请教:"敢问您服的是何种仙药?"女子言道:"这是一味中草药。知道它,它便是个宝;不知道它,它就是棵草。"

On hearing this, the "old China hand" was even more astonished and curious. He bowed and asked, "What magic medicine do you take?" The girl answered, "It's just a kind of herbal medicine. It's a treasure for one who knows it but grass for one who doesn't."

"中国通"见女子不肯轻易透露,忙匍身跪拜道:"我是波斯国王的使者,国王年老体弱,命令我带商队来贵国换一些延年益寿的中草药。我愿以全部货物换取您的草药。希望您能满足我的愿望。"

Knowing that she would not readily reveal the secret, the "old China hand" immediately kneeled down and appealed, "I'm a messenger sent by the king of Persia, who is old and feeble but hungers for longevity. For this reason, the king sent me here with my business team to exchange the herbs with our goods. I am willing to trade all my goods for your herbs. I hope you can satisfy my wish."

女子被使者的真诚打动了,便以实情相告:"这种草药全身是宝,它的名称随四季不同而变化,不同的季节要食用它不同的部位。春采枸杞叶,名天精草;夏采花,名长生草;秋采子,名枸杞子;冬采根,名地骨皮。乡人多长寿,都是食用此物的缘故啊。"使者听闻此言赞叹不已,把枸杞子带回了波斯。后来枸杞子传入中东和西方,在异域被誉为"东方神草"。

Impressed by his sincerity, the girl told the messenger the truth, "No part of this herb goes to waste. Both its name and its edible part vary with the four seasons: Leaves in spring, also known as lycium leave; flowers in summer, also known as scmpervivum; seeds in autumn, also known as fructus lycii; root bark in winter, also known as cortex lycii. Most of my fellow villagers are exceptionally long-lived just in consequence of taking this herb." On hearing this, the messenger was full of admiration and took this herb back to Persia. Later, fructus lycii came to the Middle East and the West from China, and was hailed as "Oriental Magic Grass".

枸杞子始载于《神农本草经》,这部典籍称枸杞子"久服坚筋骨,轻身不老,耐寒暑"。枸杞子味甘、性平,归肝肾,具有滋补肝肾、益精明目的功效,有"长寿果"的美称,是我国传统中药中的瑰宝。

The earliest text record pertaining to fructus lycii comes from *Shennong's Classic of Materia Medica*, which claims that "long-time consumption of fructus lycii strengthens muscles and bones, makes one seem agile and ageless, and helps endure cold winter or hot summer". Being sweet in taste and mild in nature, fructus lycii attributes to liver and kidney, and has long been thought to have medicinal virtues of nourishing the liver and kidney, replenishing the essence and brightening the eyes. It has always enjoyed the reputation of "Longevity Fruit", and serves as a gem in traditional Chinese materia medica.

第十七章 桂花

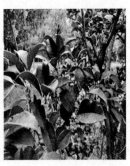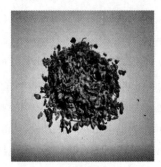

桂花

Osmanthus Fragrans

古时候,峨眉山山脚下住着一个卖酒的寡妇,她慷慨大方,菩萨心肠。由于她像西施一样貌美,酿出的酒又味道甘醇,人们就称她为"仙酒西施"。

Chapter 17　Osmanthus Fragrans

In ancient times, there lived a generous and kind-hearted widow at the foot of Mount Emei in southwest China's Sichuan Province. Her good looks run parallel to Xishi(one of the famous Four Beauties of ancient China). Being a good wine-maker, she could make perfect wine, and hence was known as the "Wine Beauty Xishi".

一年冬天,天降鹅毛大雪,寒风凛冽,天寒地冻。一大早,"仙酒西施"刚打开大门,就见一个骨瘦如柴、衣衫褴褛的年轻男子躺在地上。"仙酒西施"摸摸那人的口鼻,尚有气息,就把他背回家里,先灌热汤,又灌了杯酒,那男子渐渐舒缓过来。他感激地说:"谢谢娘子救命之恩。我无家可归,出去不是冻死,就是饿死,您发发善心,再收留我几日吧。"

On one freezing winter morning, snowflakes whirled in the sky like a myriad of feathers and a piercing cold wind kept howling. When "Wine Beauty Xishi" opened her gate, she found a scrawny young man in shabby clothes lying on the ground. Touching his mouth and nose, she found that he was still alive. She then carried him home. After drinking some hot soup and wine, the man came back to life gradually. He said gratefully, "Thank you for saving my life. But I'm homeless. I would be frozen or starve to death if I got out of this house. Please be kind, and take me in for a few days."

"仙酒西施"这下为难了,俗话说"寡妇门前是非多",像这样的年轻男子住在家中,只会招来闲言碎语。可是她转念一想,总不能眼睁睁看着他活活冻死、饿死吧!于是她点头答应,留他暂住。

The "Wine Beauty Xishi" felt awkward. As the old saying goes, "Widows are prone to invite trouble to themselves." Taking him in will only bring gossip to her, but on second thoughts she changed her mind. How could she stand by and see him die under her roof? Finally she nodded, allowing for a temporary residence.

不出所料,关于"仙酒西施"的流言蜚语很快传开了,大家开始对她敬而远之,到酒店来买酒的人越来越少。"仙酒西施"忍着内心的煎熬,依旧尽心尽力照顾那男子。后来,再也没有人来光顾她的小店,她实在无法维持生计,那男子也就不辞而别了。"仙酒西施"担心他的安危,四处寻找。

As expected, the gossip spread quickly. People started to stay at a respectful distance from her and fewer and fewer people came to buy her wine. The "Wine Beauty Xishi", however, had been enduring the suffering of her heart and taking good care of the man as usual. Over time nobody came to buy her wine and she couldn't make ends meet. One day, the man took a sudden leave without saying goodbye. It was so hard for the "Wine Beauty Xishi" to put this down that she was looking around for him.

一日,她在峨眉山上遇见一位身材瘦小的白发老翁,正挑着一担干柴,费力地向前走着。"仙酒西施"正想上前帮忙,那老人突然跌倒在地,干柴散落得到处都是。老人双目紧闭,嘴唇翕动着发出微弱的声音:"水,水……"可这荒郊野岭人迹罕至,哪来的水呢?"仙酒西施"灵机一动,咬破手指,鲜血顺着手指流了下来,她把手指伸到老人嘴边,老人瞬间消失了。一阵风刮过,穿过山谷。从天空飘下来一个布袋,布袋里装着桂花树的种子和一张纸条,上面有寥寥数语:"月宫赐丹桂,吴刚助善者。""仙酒西施"这才恍然大悟,原来那年轻男子和担柴老翁,皆是吴刚变化而来。

One day, "Wine Beauty Xishi" encountered a thin, white-haired old man who was walking forward arduously with a bunch of firewood on his shoulder on Mount Emei. As she was just about to lend a hand, the old man suddenly fell down on the ground and the firewood scattered here and there. The old man closed his eyes, moved his lips, and whispered in a low voice, "Water, water…." But how could she find water in the untraversed wilderness? On a sudden inspiration, the "Wine Beauty Xishi" broke her finger with her teeth and reached to the old man's lips with the blood trickling from her finger. At that moment the old man disappeared instantly. A gust of wind came, funneling down the valley. A cloth bag in which there were many seeds of osmanthus tree and a piece of paper was drifting down from the sky. The paper read, "It's a gift from the palace of the moon and Wu Gang is ready to help and award those well-doers." It was until then the "Wine Beauty Xishi" was suddenly enlightened that both the young man and the old man were all the embodiment of Wu Gang.

消息很快传开了,大家都争相索取桂花树的种子。心地善良的人播种下这种子,种子很快就长成一株桂花树,到了开花时节,花香沁人心脾。而心术不正的人播种下这种子,种子则不会生根发芽,这样会使他倍感蒙羞而一心向善。大家看到"仙酒西施"的时候,眼神里明显流露着敬佩之情,是她的善举打动了月宫里掌管桂花树的吴刚大仙,才把桂花种子洒向人间,从此桂花和桂花酒走进了千家万户。

The news spread quickly. People from every corner came and asked for seeds of osmanthus tree. If the kind-hearted person sowed the seeds, they would grow into trees bloomed with sweet fragrance in the yards during the flowering season. While the tree didn't even sprout in the yard if the seeds were planted by a wicked person. In this way, wicked person would be shameful and obtained a chance for renewal. People's eyes showed open admiration as they looked at "Wine Beauty Xishi". It was her good deeds that moved Wu Gang, who was in charge of the osmanthus tree in the Moon Palace and awarded the seeds to the world, thus thousands of households could enjoy both the sweet-scented osmanthus and the wine made from them.

桂花是一种天然药材。桂花味辛、性温,它的花、果、根皆可入药,具有散寒破结、化痰止咳的作用,能治牙痛、咳喘痰多和经闭腹痛等多种疾病。

Pungent in taste and warm in nature, osmanthus fragrans is a natural herb. Its flower, fruit and root can all be used as medicine with the properties of dispelling coldness, dispersing stagnation, reducing phlegm and suppressing cough. It plays a role in treating diseases such as toothache, cough and asthma with profuse phlegm, amenorrhea and abdominal pain.

第七篇　中国古代医学伦理道德

　　西晋哲学家杨泉在其《物理论》中明确指出："夫医者，非仁爱之士不可托也，非聪明达理不可任也，非廉洁淳良不可信也。"北宋刘恕所撰《通鉴外纪》记载："古者民有疾病，未知药石，炎帝始味草木之滋。……尝一日而遇七十毒，神而代之，遂作方书，以疗民疾，而医道立矣。"所谓"医道立"，就是医学伦理道德基本精神的确立：不顾个人利益安危，千方百计救死扶伤。

Section 7　Medical Ethics in Ancient China

　　As stated in *Discussion on Material Mechanisms* by philosopher Yang Quan of the Western Jin Dynasty, "As for medical practitioners, people with no benevolence and humanity cannot be entrusted, with no intelligence and reasonableness cannot be appointed, and with no clean hands and honesty seems to us to be totally unreliable and untrustworthy." According to *Tongjian Waiji*, a book compiled by Liu Shu in the Northern Song Dynasty, "In ancient times, people failed to manage herbal remedies when they got sick. Therefore, Shennong began to taste many kinds of herbs daily to determine which could be used for curing diseases.... In this practice he once was poisoned by 70 toxic herbs in a day but was out of danger by drinking tea. Hence he compiled medical formulary to help sick people, and medical ethics was established accordingly." By "medical ethics" we mean the establishment of the basic spirit of it: TCM practitioners make every attempt to heal the wounded and rescue the dying regardless of individual interest or safety, and personal gains or losses.

第一章 大医精诚

《大医精诚》一文出自唐朝孙思邈所著《备急千金要方》第一卷,乃是中医典籍中论述医德的一篇极其重要的文献,为习医者所必读。《大医精诚》认为习医之人不仅要有精湛的医术,还要拥有良好的医德。这篇文章广为流传,影响深远。直到现在,我国的不少中医院校仍将它作为医学誓言,并把它当作行为准则来严格要求自己。《大医精诚》被誉为"东方的希波克拉底誓言"。原文如下:

Chapter 1 On the Absolute Sincerity of Great Doctors

The article *On the Absolute Sincerity of Great Doctors* comes from the first volume of *Prescriptions Worth a Thousand Pieces of Gold for Emergencies* by Sun Simiao in the Tang Dynasty of China. It is a must-read for TCM practitioners for it is a highly important document on medical ethics in classics of TCM. This article, spreading from mouth to mouth, raises a twofold necessary qualification for TCM practitioners, to possess superb medical skills and to own lofty medical ethics, exerting far-reaching impact. Until now there has been a trickle of TCM universities which adopt it as a classical Chinese medicine oath and make it the code of conduct to hold oneself with strictness. This classic is hailed as "Eastern Hippocratic Oath". Its original appearance goes as follows:

凡大医治病,必当安神定志,无欲无求,先发大慈恻隐之心,誓愿普救含灵之苦。若有疾厄来求救者,不得问其贵贱贫富,长幼妍蚩,怨亲善友,华夷愚智,普同一等,皆如至亲之想。亦不得瞻前顾后,自虑吉凶,护惜身命。见彼苦恼,若己有之,深心凄怆。勿避险巇、昼夜、寒暑、饥渴、疲劳,一心赴救,无作功夫形迹之心。如此可为苍生大医,反此则是含灵巨贼。自古名贤治病,多用生命以济危急,虽曰贱畜贵人，至于爱命，人畜一也。损彼益己，物情同患，况于人乎。夫杀生求生，去生更远。吾今此方，所以不用生命为药者，良由此也。其虻虫、水蛭之属，市有先死者，则市而用之，不在此例。只如鸡卵一物，以其混沌未分，必有大段要急之处，不得已隐忍而用之。能不用者，斯为大哲亦所不及也。其有患疮痍下痢，臭秽不可瞻视，人所恶见者，但发惭愧、凄怜、忧恤之意，不得起一念蒂芥之心，是吾之志也。

Any great doctor who cures the sickness will deservedly calm down, settle his mind and desire for nothing. Overflowing with the milk of human kindness, he first vows to relieve hardships of the people under heaven. If the patients come to seek help, he should act fairly to all of them and hold them as very close relatives, regardless of their status, wealth, age, appearance, affinity, nationality and education. He may not be overcautious, nor does he look before and behind, worry about personal gains and losses and cherish his own life. Seeing the patients' bitter struggle, he regards their sufferings as his own and has deep sympathy for them. Being wrapped up in healing the wounded and rescuing the dying, he not only forgets difficulties and dangers, day and night, cold and heat, hunger and thirst, tiredness and drowsiness, but also leaves superficial practice and surface acting far behind him. Only in this way can he become a great doctor. Otherwise, he will approach an end to sleaze. Since ancient times, prestigious doctors mostly used living creatures to rescue patients in desperate situations. Although livestock are believed to be inferior to noble humans, they are the same as for treasuring life. To kill one for the rescue of another is deemed to be a sad case of cruelty even in the animal world, let alone human beings! Seeking the survival of mankind by killing animals actually deviates from the doctor's original aspiration of saving lives. This is why the prescriptions recorded in my book have excluded the use of living creatures. Creatures such as gadfly, leech and the like will be an exception if they are already dead before being sold on the market. If so, then we can buy them with a medical purpose. What makes the egg so special is that it is still in a chaotic undivided situation and has not become a chick. Hence it can only be used under emergency as a last resort. Those who can handle without the use of eggs are real great doctors without parallel. Sometimes patients are suffering from scabies, sore or dysentery which causes people to shrink away from the sufferers due to the funky odors and unpleasant appearances. But as a doctor, the sight of it should provoke the feelings of shame, compassion and mercy instead of giving them a cold shoulder. This is my ambition spurring me on.

孙思邈的医学伦理观在中医药史上非常重要。他在《备急千金要方》中首次提出了"大医精诚"的概念，对医生必须遵循的医学道德指导原则进行了全面的论述。他认为"人命至重，有贵千金，一方济之，德逾于此"，他的书名为《备急千金要方》，就是这种高尚道德品格的体现。历代讲医德者，无不首先提到这篇文章，它至今仍有重要的教育意义。

Sun Simiao's viewpoint on medical ethics is of great significance in the history of TCM. In his *Prescriptions Worth a Thousand Pieces of Gold for Emergencies*, the notion of "the Absolute Sincerity of Great Doctors" was first proposed, offering a full-scale elaboration to the guiding principles of medical ethics a doctor must stick to. He deems that "Human life is the most important, and it is more precious than a thousand pieces of gold. Nothing could be more virtuous than to save life with one prescription." His book is entitled *Prescriptions Worth a Thousand Pieces of Gold for Emergencies*, which is just a manifestation of such noble moral character. When it comes to medical ethics, it is only natural that invariably this article will be first mentioned throughout the ages. It still has great educational significance now.

第二章　悬壶济世

中国人有句俗语，那就是"葫芦里不知卖的什么药"。这个典故出自南朝范晔所著《后汉书》："市中有一老翁，悬一壶于肆头。及市罢，辄跳入壶中。市人莫之见，惟长房于楼上睹之，异焉。因往再拜，奉酒脯。翁知长房之意其神也，谓之曰：'子明日可更来。'长房旦日复诣翁，翁乃与俱入壶中。惟见玉堂严丽，旨酒甘肴，盈衍其中。共饮毕而出。后长房欲求道，随从入山。翁抚之曰：'子可教也。'遂可医疗众疾。"

Chapter 2　Hanging a Bottle-Gourd to Benefit all Mankind

As the Chinese saying goes, "What medicine does he sell in his bottle-gourd?" This classical allusion comes from *The Book of the Later Han Dynasty* by Fan Ye during the Southern Dynasties. "There was once an old man selling medicine in a market with a bottle-gourd hanging in front of his stall. Whenever the market closed, he would jump into the bottle-gourd. No one in the market noticed it except Fei Zhangfang, a petty official managing the market. He stared in wonder at the entire scene. Therefore, he came to visit the old man, presenting wine and dried meat. Knowing that Fei had elevated him to godlike status, the old man invited him to come here tomorrow. The next day, Fei paid the old man another visit and both of them jumped into the bottle-gourd. Fei caught a glimpse of the magnificent palace and the whole table of good wine and dainty dishes. They drank to their hearts' content and walked out of the bottle-gourd. Later, Fei intended to study medicine and so he lived in seclusion with the old man. The old man stroked Fei gently and said, 'You are worth teaching.' Fei then acquired the skill which enabled him to cure various diseases."

"悬壶"这一典故,葛洪在其《神仙传》中亦有类似的记载,这就是"悬壶"的由来。所以后人把行医称为"悬壶",而悬挂的葫芦就成了中医的标志。

Similar records of "Hanging a Bottle-Gourd" can be found in *Biographies of Immortals* by Ge Hong. This is the origin of the classical allusion "Hanging a Bottle-Gourd". Hence later generations call practising medicine "Hanging a Bottle-Gourd", and the hanging bottle-gourd has become the hallmark of TCM.

第三章　杏林春暖

"杏林春暖"的典故广泛流传于中医学界。"杏林"一词源自三国时期的名医董奉的故事。董奉和当时南阳的张仲景、谯郡的华佗并称为"建安三神医"。

Chapter 3　Apricot Orchard in the Warmth of Spring

The literary quotation "Apricot Orchard in the Warmth of Spring" has been widely circulated in TCM profession. The term "Apricot Orchard" originated from the story of Dong Feng, a distinguished doctor during the Three Kingdoms Period. Zhang Zhongjing, a famous medical scientist from Nanyang, together with Hua Tuo from Qiao County and Dong Feng became known as the "Three Highly Skilled Doctors during the Jian'an Period" at that time.

据葛洪的《神仙传》记载,董奉是三国时期东吴侯官人。董奉四处巡诊,后来回到南昌,就在庐山定居了下来。董奉住在山上却不种田,每日为人治病,分文不取。如果重病的病人被治愈了,他就让病人栽种五棵杏树;如果是轻症的病人被治好了,他就让病人栽种一棵杏树。如此数年,栽种了十万余棵杏树,这些杏树郁然成林。杏林山中的百禽群兽都在杏树之下游戏,杏林一年到头杂草不生,就像有人经常锄耕管理一样。

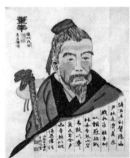

董奉像
Portrait of Dong Feng

According to *Biographies of Immortals* by Ge Hong, Dong Feng, was a native of Houguan County of the Eastern Wu Kingdom in the Three Kingdoms Period. As a doctor,

Dong Feng made his rounds of visits everywhere. Later, he settled in Lushan Mountain when he went back to Nanchang City. Dong Feng lived in the mountain but didn't do farming. Day after day he cared for patients without any charge. If a patient with a serious disease got cured, Dong Feng would ask him to plant five apricot trees; for a patient with slight illness, one apricot tree was enough. Several years passed, more than 100,000 green and luxuriant apricot trees made an orchard with numerous birds and beasts in the mountain sporting under the apricot trees. All the year round the apricot orchard was free from any weeds, and it seemed as though it was in constant cultivation and management.

后来，所种之杏大量成熟，董奉就在杏林里搭建一个草仓储杏，以便告知世人：欲买杏者，不必告诉我，只要往粮仓里放入一些谷子，就可以自己取走相同分量的杏。曾经有人放入的谷子少而取走的杏多，杏林里便有群虎吼叫追逐，那人十分惶恐，急忙提着杏顺着路旁逃跑，不料杏撒了一地。到家后，那人一看，拿回来的杏竟和送去的谷子一样多。有时有人偷杏，老虎就追到他家，直到把他咬死。他的家人知道偷杏的事情后，就把偷来的杏如数奉还，叩头谢过，董奉才又使其复活。董奉每年用杏换得谷子，以此来救济贫困者，供给行旅之资不足者，每年救济多达两万余人。

Later, when large quantities of apricots were ripe, Dong Feng built a straw storehouse in the orchard to store apricots and inform the local people, "Anyone who wants to buy apricots needs to put some grains in the straw storehouse and can take the same amount of apricots without telling me." There were people who took more than they gave. Once found, the tigers in the orchard would snarl at and chase after them. Once a man was terrified and tried to escape hastily with the apricots along the roadside, but he scattered the apricots all over the ground. After arriving home, he weighed the apricots, only to find that the remains of the apricots were the exact amount he should have taken. Whenever pilfering occurred, tigers in the orchard would follow the thief and bite him to death. After knowing all this, his family would then return the apricots and kneel down to apologize for his wrongdoing.

Dong Feng then tried to revive him. Every year, Dong Feng exchanged apricots for grains in order to relieve poverty-stricken families and assist travelers who ran out of supplies. The total tally of relief surpassed 20,000 people each year.

董奉的故事被后世传为佳话,"杏林"成了中医学界的雅称,"杏林春暖"成了中医药行业的代名词和人们最喜欢用的成语之一。人们常用"杏林春暖""杏林春满"等成语来称颂医德高尚、医术精湛的医生,把医术高明的医生称为"杏林高手",把和中医药有关的故事叫作"杏林佳话"。

The story of Dong Feng has become a much-told tale and "*Xinglin*" (Apricot Orchard) has become a kind of elegant name of the TCM community. "*Xinglin Chunnuan*" (Apricot Orchard in the Warmth of Spring) has turned into a byword for TCM profession and one of the most popular idioms. Idioms such as "*Xinglin Chunnuan*" (Apricot Orchard in the Warmth of Spring) and "*Xinglin Chunman*" (Apricot Orchard in All the World's Spring) are frequently used to extol doctors with noble medical ethics and superb medical skills. A highly skilled doctor comes to be known as the "*Xinglin Gaoshou*" (An Expert in TCM) and stories relevant to TCM are referred to as "*Xinglin Jiahua*" (Stories Associated with TCM on Everybody's Lips).

第四章　橘井泉香

"橘井泉香"的典故出自西汉刘向所撰《列仙传》之《苏耽传》。苏耽,湖南郴州人,西汉文帝时,他熟谙养生之道,人称苏仙。苏耽幼年丧父,以孝顺母亲著闻乡里。他家住县城东北,离城有一百余里。有一天,苏耽与母亲正在进食,母亲对他说:"没有腌鱼啊。"苏耽立刻放下筷子,起身取钱离去。片刻间,他就拿着腌鱼回来了。母亲问他:"从何处得来的?"苏耽回答道:"县城里买的。"母亲说:"从家到县城往返百余里,顷刻而至,你是在骗我呀!"苏耽对母亲说:"买鱼的时候,遇见了舅父,与舅父约定,明天到咱家来。"第二天,苏耽的舅父果然如期而至。

Chapter 4　Tangerine Leaves and Well Water

The allusion "Tangerine Leaves and Well Water" stems from the chapter *Biographies of Su Dan* in *Biographies of Immortals* by Liu Xiang in the Western Han Dynasty. Su Dan, a native of Chenzhou County, Hunan Province, was known as an immortal for he had been well versed in ways of keeping good health during the period of Emperor Wen of Han. When Su Dan was very young, his father died. Su Dan was known for his filial piety to his mother throughout the neighbourhood. He lived in the northeast of Chenzhou County, which was more than a hundred miles from town. One day, while having meal, his mother said that they had run out of salted fish. Su Dan put down his chopsticks at once, took some money and went out. Within moments, he came back with a salted fish. His mother asked him, "Where did you get it?" He responded that he bought it from the county town. "It's over a hundred miles from home to the county town, how can you come back in a blink of an eye? You must be fooling me!" exclaimed his mother. Su Dan said to his mother, "I came across my uncle when I bought fish. We agreed to meet at our home tomorrow." The next day, his uncle did come as expected.

有一天,天上的仪仗队从空中飘然降落至苏宅。苏耽对母亲说:"我已受命将名字载入神仙簿籍了,今日便要离家而去,不能再奉养母亲了。"苏耽的母亲说:"我何以存活?"苏耽留下两个盘子,母亲需要饮食就敲小盘,需要钱帛就敲大盘,所需之物立即送到。

One day, a guard of honour floated down to his home from the sky. Su Dan said to his mother, "I have been appointed to have my name forever be tied to the register of immortals. Today I am about to leave, and can't support and wait upon you any longer." "How can I survive on my own?" said his mother. Su Dan told his mother he would leave her two plates. She might knock at the smaller one for food, and the bigger one for money or textiles. Daily necessities would be served immediately.

苏耽又对母亲说:"明年天下将有一场瘟疫,院子里的井水和橘树能够治疗此病。凡是染上疫病的人,给他一升井水,一片橘叶,煎汤饮服,立即痊愈。"后来,果然发生疫病,远至千里的人都来求井水橘叶,饮服井水橘叶者,即刻痊愈。

"An epidemic will break out next year." Su Dan informed his mother. "The well water and the tangerine tree in the yard can deal with such disease. Anyone who is struck by the epidemic may get a liter of well water and a tangerine leaf. The sufferer will be fine immediately once he or she decocts the tangerine leaf in the well water and drinks it all." Later, an epidemic really broke out. The sufferers took the trouble of travelling a thousand miles to obtain the well water and the tangerine leaves. One who drank the decoction would heal in no time.

从此,"橘井"一词逐渐演化为中医药的代名词,人们以"橘井泉香"来称颂行医者治病救人的功绩。"橘井泉香"和"悬壶济世""杏林春暖"一起,成为中医学界脍炙人口的三大典故。

Since then, the term "*Tangerine and Well*" also gradually evolved into an equivalent for TCM. "Tangerine Leaves and Well Water" has been used to extol the merits and achievements of TCM practitioners ever since. "Tangerine Leaves and Well Water", together with "Hanging a Bottle-Gourd to Benefit All Mankind" and "Apricot Orchard in the Warmth of Spring" have become three most popular classical allusions on everybody's lips in TCM circles.

第五章　诊宗三昧

明末清初,一代名医张璐在其所著《诊宗三昧·宗旨》中向当世行医之人提出了三大警醒:其一,有些医生凭借家传世医的名声,抱技通神,止步不前,株守家传,任意抛却、剔除岐黄之术,不顾医学的本源,这些做法都是因为他们不谙行医之道。其二,有些医生弃儒学而行医,只知道博览医书却没有完整的师传。用药时只知道一味地温补且极力抵制苦寒之药,这些做法都是因为他们不通权变。其三,有些医生欺世盗名,结交能言善辩但心术不正之人,凭借声名攀附权贵,大张旗鼓地炫耀自己的医术,曲意逢迎世风世俗,治死无辜,敛财果腹,竭尽心力博家人一笑,这些做法都是因为他们医德沦丧。

Chapter 5　Three Warnings in Practising Medicine

Zhang Lu, a distinguished doctor in the late Ming and early Qing Dynasty, once put forward three warnings sharply in practising medicine at that time in his book *Three Warnings in Practising Medicine*.

First, some doctors counted on reputation handed down from a family for generations, carried incomparable hidden talents and skills, ceased to advance a step further, held on medical skills handed down from the older generations of the family stubbornly, discarded and rejected Chinese herbal medical science at will and ignored the ultimate source of medical science, all of which resulted from their ignorance of the ways of practising medicine.

Second, some doctors cast aside Confucianism and went into practising medicine. Instead of achieving an intact succession of teachings from a master to his disciples, they only knew how to browse medical books extensively. While giving medication, they blindly preferred warm-tonification drugs to those bitter and cold in nature, all of which derived from a lack of flexibility and adaptability.

Third, some doctors angled for undeserved fame, associated with those who were eloquent but harbored evil intentions, and played up to people of power and influence on the strength of reputation. Besides, they flaunted their medical skills with colors flying and the band playing, flattered common practice of society and common customs in a hundred and one ways. What's more, they put the innocent patients to death due to incompetence, accumulated wealth by unfair means to fill the stomach, and exerted their hearts and strength to the utmost just for a smile of their families. All these behaviors were exactly the source of medical ethics collapse.

这篇文章言辞犀利、鞭辟入里、发人深省,至今仍有借鉴意义。

This article, which is trenchant, penetrating and thought-provoking, reflects the author's views, and is by now of great referential significance.

第六章　不为良相，愿为良医

据南宋吴曾《能改斋漫录》记载，北宋著名政治家、文学家范仲淹低微贫贱之时，曾经到寺庙里向神灵祷告："他日能得宰相之位吗？"神灵不语。范仲淹又祷告说："不能得相位，愿为良医。"神灵亦不语。范仲淹随后感叹说："不能为百姓谋利造福，这并非大丈夫平生的志向。"

Chapter 6　Be a Good Prime Minister, or Be a Good Doctor

According to *Casual Records of Nenggai Study* by Wu Zeng of the Southern Song Dynasty (1127 A.D.–1279 A.D.), when Fan Zhongyan, a renowned Song Dynasty politician and writer, was humble, poor and lowly, he once went to a temple and prayed, "Will I get the position of prime minister in the future?" There was no response. He then prayed again, "If I can't be a good prime minister to help govern the country, I would like to be a good doctor to save lives." There was still no answer. "One who fails to labour assiduously for the benefit of ordinary people deviates from the ambition of a true man." sighed Fan Zhongyan.

有一天，有人对范仲淹说："大丈夫立志当宰相是理所当然的，而医术再高明也只是一门技艺而已，您为什么愿意如此呢？这样是不是太卑微了？"

One day, someone asked Fan, "It ought to go without saying that a true man should aspire to be a prime minister. The profession of medicine is nothing but technique. Why are you willing to be a doctor? This is so humble, isn't it？"

范仲淹回答说:"哎呀! 难道是为了这些吗? 宰相固然可以恩及天下百姓,然而当不能得到相位时,能救助百姓、为天下谋取利益的,没有什么能比得上良医了。果真能成为良医的话,上可以治疗国君和双亲的疾病,下可以缓解黎民百姓的病痛,除此之外,还可以保养自己的身体,使自己长久健康。处下位而能恩及天下百姓的,也唯有良医能做到了。"

"Oh! It is for these? No doubt a prime minister can bestow favors to people. But when one fails to get this position, there's nothing better than to be a doctor to assist the ordinary people and benefit the world. If so, he can cure not only monarch and parents, but also ordinary people. What's more, he can take care of his own body and live healthily for as long as possible. No other profession allows one to favor ordinary people when in a low position." Fan Zhongyan replied.

这则历史琐闻记述了范仲淹年轻时"不为良相,愿为良医"的抱负。这就是后世相传"不为良相,愿为良医"的由来。"不为良相,愿为良医"早已成为中国古代医家的座右铭。

This historical scrap of information unfolds before our eyes the ambition of Fan Zhongyan in his youth. That's where the quotation "Be a Good Prime Minister, or Be a Good Doctor" passed down through the generations came from. Such a quotation has long been regarded as a motto of medical practitioners in ancient China.

第八篇　中医千年抗疫史

回望中华民族的历史,中医和疫病的抗争从未停止过。人类的文明史,在很大程度上就是一部不断与疫病抗争的历史。在与疫病抗争的几千年历史中,中医从未缺席,均积极参与其中并发挥了独特的治疗优势。

Section 8　TCM Fighting Epidemic with Thousands of Years' History

Looking back at the history of Chinese nation, TCM's fight against the epidemic has never stopped. The history of human civilization has been, to a large extent, a history of constant struggle with anti-epidemic fight. TCM, which has a recorded history of anti-epidemic stretching back over thousands of years, has never been absent from the battle, but has joined early and participated actively, displaying its unique strengths in preventing and treating epidemic diseases.

第一章　先秦时期

关于疫病,人类很早就对其有相关的认识。中国最早的相关文字记载源自商朝。早在三千多年前,河南安阳殷墟出土的甲骨文便有"疾年"以及"疥、疟、首风"等传染病名称的记载。不仅如此,在甲骨文中还有"寇扫"的记载,反映出古人已经意识到保持环境卫生对于防疫的重要性。

Chapter 1　Pre-Qin Period

With regard to epidemic disease, mankind gained relevant recognition of it a long time ago. The earliest written records in China, whose links with epidemic disease dated back to the Shang Dynasty, were found on the oracle bone inscriptions unearthed at the 3,300-year-old Yinxu Ruins in Anyang, Henan Province. A trace of earliest recorded "epidemic-prone year" was found, indicating that people were more prone to catch epidemic diseases in that year, and an abundance of records such as scabies, malaria and head-wind syndrom were used to describe the names of epidemic diseases. Records of thorough household cleaning reflected that the ancients had already realized the magnitude of keeping the environment clean.

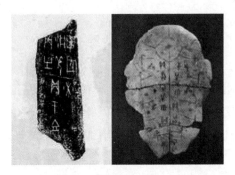

甲骨文

Oracle Bone Inscriptions

中国奇书《山海经》中不仅有占卜"天下大疫"的记录,也有关于"疫、疠、疟、疥"的记载。古人认识到保持良好的环境卫生和个人卫生有助于防止感染疫病,《山海经》还提出人畜分居、房屋清扫、除虫洗澡等保持卫生的措施。

The ever recorded divination practising of "large outbreak of epidemic under heaven" came from a fascinating Chinese book *The Classic of Mountains and Seas*, in which epidemic, catastrophic malignant disease, malaria and scabies also had been well documented. The ancients gained an increase in awareness that environmental health and personal hygiene helped prevent catching epidemic diseases. *The Classic of Mountains and Seas* raised a set of epidemic prevention measures such as human and livestock separation, cleaning the house, disinsectization and taking a bath, etc.

据1975年在湖北省云梦县睡虎地秦墓中出土的《睡虎地秦墓竹简》记载,我国秦朝时期已经建立了疫情报告制度。在《睡虎地秦墓竹简·法律问答》中,首次出现了"疠所"一词。"疠所"就是专门用来隔离传染病患者的地方,开创了我国传染病隔离制度设立的先河。据《睡虎地秦墓竹简·毒言》记载,知情者应断绝与患"毒言"(一种颇具危害的传染病)者的接触。

According to *Shuihudi Bamboo Slips of the Qin Dynasty* excavated from the tomb in Yunmeng County, Hubei Province, landmark discoveries included the establishment of the direct reporting system for epidemic erupts in the Qin Dynasty. As stated in *Shuihudi Bamboo Slips of the Qin Dynasty: Reply for the Legal Enquiry*, the term "Quarantine Sites", which was coined for the first time and literally meant quarantine area exclusively for those suffering from infectious diseases, undoubtedly pioneered the establishment of the quarantine system for infectious diseases in China. Records from *Shuihudi Bamboo Slips of the Qin Dynasty: Duyan* showed that the rules coming into force at that time bolstered insiders' cutting off ties with people who had developed *duyan* (a kind of hazardous infectious disease).

我国最早的中医经典著作《黄帝内经》中就不乏关于疫病的相关论述。第9卷《黄帝内经·素问·评热病论》明确指出了发病的原因:"邪之所凑,其气必虚。"第21卷中《黄帝内经·素问·六元正纪大论》有"厉大至,民善暴死"的论述,指出"疠"是具有极强传染性的疾病。"其病温厉大行,远近咸若。"这说明疫病发生时,无论男女老少,所有人都是易感人群。

Epidemic diseases are also recorded in *Inner Canon of the Yellow Emperor*, the greatest and oldest Chinese medical classic, which is packed to the brim with some related discussions. In volume 9, *Plain Questions: Comment on Febrile Diseases* makes clear that "Accumulation of evil *qi* will inevitably lead to deficiency of vital healthy *qi*", which explains the causes of diseases. In volume 21, *Plain Questions: Major Discussion on the Progress of the Six Climatic Changes* has some observations on the highly contagious disease *li* (catastrophic malignant disease), "The prevalence of pestilence tends to cause sudden death, warm disease and pestilence were becoming prevalent on parallel tracks and people suffered from the same diseases, whether near or far away." This suggests that all people without exception are vulnerable to epidemic diseases when they occur.

《黄帝内经》中确立的扶正祛邪的防疫基本思想体现在第 21 卷《黄帝内经·素问·刺法论》黄帝和岐伯的一段对话中：

The basic idea of strengthening the healthy vital *qi* and eliminating the pathogenic evil *qi* established in *Inner Canon of the Yellow Emperor* is recorded in a conversation around anti-epidemic fight presented by the mythological Yellow Emperor and Qi Bo in volume 21, *Plain Questions: Discussion on Acupuncture Methods*.

黄帝曰："余闻五疫之至，皆相染易，无问大小，病状相似，不施救疗，如何可得不相移易者？"

岐伯曰："不相染者，正气存内，邪不可干；避其毒气，天牝从来，复得其往。"

Yellow Emperor remarks, "I've heard that evidence of various epidemic diseases has emerged, and there is a risk of person-to-person transmission. A large crowd of people, whether young or old, present similar symptoms. How to prevent and control the infection if there is no medical assistance?"

"Invasion of pathogenic factors will get nowhere as long as sufficient healthy vital *qi* exists inside the body. Perhaps that's why there is no infection when epidemic diseases break out." Qi Bo responded, "also measures should come to avoid potential risks of the invasion of pathogenic toxic *qi*. Pathogenic evil *qi* gets in and out of the body through the nose."

黄帝和岐伯口中的"皆相染易""病状相似""避其毒气""天牝从来"等疫病特征与今天的疫病特征如出一辙。

There is undoubtedly a great deal of epidemic disease characteristics following the same track with today's pandemic in what Yellow Emperor and Qi Bo unveiled : "a risk of person-to-person transmission" "similar symptoms" "measures to avoid pathogenic toxic *qi*" "source of infection coming from respiratory system".

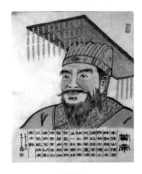 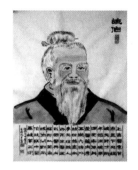

黄帝　　　　　　　岐伯
Yellow Emperor　　Qi Bo

《黄帝内经》明确指出,疫病的感染与人体内的正气有密切关系。正气充足,则外邪不侵;正气虚弱,则百邪丛生,故而引发疾病。由此可见,在疫病防治上须注重扶正祛邪,增强人体的正气,如此才能够如《黄帝内经·素问·上古天真论第一》所讲的那样,"精神内守,病安从来"。除了"正气存内,邪不可干"的防疫观,《黄帝内经》还提出了"不治已病治未病"的防治观,这种未病先防的指导原则已被证实是有效的预防传染病的方法。

The risk of infection with epidemic diseases correlates closely with the state of healthy vital *qi*. This was clearly articulated in *Inner Canon of the Yellow Emperor*, which claims that sufficiency of healthy vital *qi* bolsters the body's defence against the diseases, while deficiency of healthy vital *qi* causes various pathogenic factors, triggering the invasion of diseases. With the importance of strengthening the healthy vital *qi* and eliminating the pathogenic evil *qi* self-evident in the context of prevention and treatment of diseases, beefing up healthy vital *qi* helps the body resist infection. Only in this way can "essence-spirit remaining inside without any loss and disease finding no way to occur". That's what *Plain Questions*: *Ancient Ideas on How to Preserve Natural Healthy Energy* intends to convey. Besides views on fighting epidemic, this classic also raises views of "prevention first—an ounce of prevention is worth a pound of cure". This preventative guideline is clearly the effective approach in tackling the epidemic threat, which so far has been attested by medical practice.

《墨子·尚同》曰:"故当若天降寒热不节,雪霜雨露不时,五谷不孰,六畜不遂,疾灾戾疫。"《礼记·孟春之月·月令》记载:"孟春行秋令,则民大疫。"《吕氏春秋·季春纪》中也有类似的表达:"季春行夏令,则民多疾疫。"可见,古人已经认识到疫病的发生与气候、时令等有很大关系。

Records from *Mozi*: *Identifying with the Superior* states that "When cold and heat come unseasonably, likewise, snow, frost, rain and dew arrive untimely, the five grains will fail to turn ripe and the livestock grow slowly. Diseases, disasters, pestilences and epidemics come one after another." *The Book of Rites*: *During the First Month of Spring* gives the same voice, "During the first month of spring, if an untimely decree for autumn is promulgated, severe pestilence will occur." A similar belief is also recorded in *Spring and Autumn Annals of Lv Buwei*: *Records on the Third Month of the Spring Season*, "In spring, if an unseasonable and untimely decree for summer is promulgated, epidemic disease is prone to occur." It was glaringly obvious that for the ancients, climate and season made a big difference in the occurrence of pestilence.

《孟子·离娄章句下》曰:"西子蒙不洁,则人皆掩鼻而过之。"这说明古人已经意识到佩戴口罩能够阻挡细菌和有害气体的侵袭。

And the embryonic form of the mask, is known by most Chinese from the book *Mencius*: *Li Lou*, "If the body of Xishi (ancient Chinese celebrity, one of the famous Four Beauties of ancient China) is covered with filth, the passers-by will stuff up their noses with silk fabric to ward off the unpleasant odours." This shows that the ancients had already hoisted themselves into awareness of wearing masks which could block the invasion of bacteria and harmful gases.

营造卫生整洁的环境,可以筑牢防治疫情的防线。古人已有清晨起床后打扫室内外环境卫生的习惯,据《礼记》记载:"鸡初鸣……洒扫室堂及庭。"

Creating a clean and tidy environment helps cement the line of defense against epidemic disease. The ancients already had the habit of making a thorough indoor and outdoor clearing after getting up in the early morning, According to *The Book of Rites*, "People attempt to keep the house and yard tidy upon hearing the first crow of a rooster."

第二章　两汉三国时期

疫,本义为流行性急性传染病。我国历史上第一部权威字典《说文解字》对其的解释为:"疠者,恶疾也;疫者,民皆疾也。"

Chapter 2　The Han Dynasties and the Three Kingdoms Period

The original meaning of the character yi was a kind of pandemic acute infectious disease, which was defined in China's first authoritative dictionary, *Shuo Wen Jie Zi*, written by Xu Shen in the Eastern Han Dynasty, as "*Li* is a catastrophic malignant disease not yi(epidemic). When yi (epidemic) breaks out, all people without exception get sick."

西汉时期的哲学著作《淮南子》载有"猘狗不投于河",这说明古人对水源卫生的重视。

The Western Han philosophical masterpiece on ancient Chinese history, *Huainanzi*, had these words, "Rabid dog is expressly forbidden to drop into a river", which showed that the ancients placed a high value on sanitation of water sources.

西周时期的著名政治家、思想家周公旦所著《周礼·天官·冢宰》中早已有关于疫病的记载:"疾医掌养万民之疾病。四时皆有疠疾:春时有痟首疾,夏时有痒疥疾,秋时有疟寒疾,冬时有漱上气疾。"这说明古人对疫病的认知已经达到了一定的水平,认为疫病一年四季皆有可能发生。

Likewise, in ancient China, according to *Rites of Zhou*: *Officer of Heaven* by a remarkable politician and thinker named Duke of Zhou, "The physician held responsible for diseases of the masses. Epidemic diseases occurred throughout the year: headaches in spring, scabies in summer, malaria and aversion to cold in autumn, and cough and asthma in winter." These records indicated that in the early days, the ancients had not just an inkling that epidemic diseases might occur all year round, which mirrored that their cognitive level about epidemic diseases was up to scratch.

东汉著名的历史学家班固所著《汉书·平帝纪》中载有隔离预防疫病的措施:"民疾疫者,空舍邸第,为置医药。"这也是我国最早的关于公立临时时疫医院雏形的记录。据《后汉书·皇甫规传》记载,东汉名将皇甫规在陇右时,"军中大疫,死者十三四,规亲入庵庐巡视",这说明当时已经采取针对疫病设置专门隔离区"庵庐"的治疗手段,这也可以称得上是比较早的"方舱医院"了。

History of Han, works of renowned Han Dynasty historian Ban Gu, showed tightening pestilence prevention quarantine measures, "When a pestilence swept the land under the reign of the Emperor Ping, the local government requisitioned houses of the dignitaries to lodge infected people and provide medical treatment." This was the first public makeshift epidemic hospital of its kind in embryo established in China. According to ancient classic *A History of the Later Han Dynasty*: *Biography of Huangfu Gui*, "A severe pestilence spread in the barracks in Longyou, which caused the deaths of about 13 or 14 soldiers. Huangfu Gui, a famous general of the Eastern Han Dynasty, went on a tour of inspection of *anlu* (a special quarantine site in the army) personally." This said a lot that *anlu* (a special quarantine site in the army), which deserved to be called the earlier "Fangcang Makeshift Hospital" in China, served as a right implementation approach of epidemic prevention.

东汉末年,战乱频繁,瘟疫肆虐,病死了很多人。张仲景在《伤寒杂病论》序言中写道:"余宗族素多,向余二百。建安纪年以来,犹未十稔,其死亡者,三分有二,伤寒十居其七。"那时伤寒病包括霍乱、痢疾、肺炎、流行性感冒等一系列急性传染病。东汉末年,大多数医生对这种流行病束手无策,没有对症治疗的办法,诚如东汉末年曹植《说疫气》所言,成百上千的人被夺走了生命。当张仲景目击传染病肆虐屠城,很多亲属被夺去生命的惨象后,他决心攻克这种疾病。这种千门灭户的惨状直接促成了《伤寒杂病论》的诞生,其中《伤寒论》创立了六经辨证体系,论述了人体感受外邪导致外感疾病的辩证思想,为后世系统诊疗疫病奠定了基础。

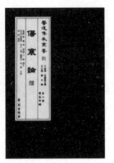 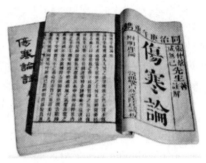

《伤寒论》
Treatise on Febrile Diseases

The late Eastern Han Dynasty was rife with war and plague which killed a lot of people. As Zhang Zhongjing stated in the preface to *Treatise on Febrile Diseases and Miscellaneous Illnesses* that "Originally my clan had more than 200 members. However, from the first year of the Jian'an reign, two thirds of them died of epidemic within ten years, of which cold-induced febrile diseases caused by cold accounted for 70 percent." Cold-induced febrile disease at that time involved cholera, dysentery, pneumonia, flu and some other acute infectious diseases. In the last years of Eastern Han Dynasty, most doctors were at the end of their resources because there was certainly no cure for such diseases. As stated in *A Discussion on Epidemic Disease* by Cao Zhi during the late Eastern Han

Dynasty, consequently, the prevalent pestilence claimed the lives of hundreds of thousands of people. Zhang Zhongjing determined to conquer this disease after he witnessed the pitiful sight of epidemic ravaging his city and killing most of his relatives. Such pitiful sight of destruction of a thousand families was the midwife to the birth of *Treatise on Febrile Diseases and Miscellaneous Illnesses*, among which *Treatise on Febrile Diseases* created six-meridian syndrome differentiation system centering around the dialectical thought of exogenous diseases resulting from exogenous pathogenic factors, thus laying the groundwork for future diagnosis and treatment of epidemic diseases.

第三章 魏晋南北朝时期

东晋葛洪的《肘后备急方》中首次记录了"虏疮"(天花)和"沙虱病"(恙虫病)的症状和治疗方药。此书还载有"狂犬咬"(狂犬病)、"虏黄病"(钩端螺旋体病)等多种传染性疾病及其治疗方法。他在《肘后备急方》中所记载"疗猘犬咬人方……仍杀所咬犬,取脑敷之,后不复发"的中医防治狂犬病免疫技术方面的经验,体现了"以毒攻毒"的免疫学思想,被认为是中国免疫思想的萌芽,为世界免疫学做出了贡献。

Chapter 3 Period of the Wei, Jin, and Southern and Northern Dynasties

During the Eastern Jin Dynasty, in Ge Hong's *Handbook of Prescriptions for Emergencies*, it claimed its first record of symptoms and treatment prescriptions for smallpox and tsutsugamushi disease (chigger) in the world. It also documented many other infectious diseases such as hydrophobia, leptospirosis and the corresponding therapies. In this book, he wrote that "There was prescription serving as remedy for dog bites…no signs of a relapse was showing after killing the biting dog and applying its brain to the bites." In terms of prevention and treatment of hydrophobia with TCM, the remarkable experience in such accumulated immunological technique, which was known as the embryos of immune thought, reflected the immunological thought of "combating poison with poison", and truly contributed to immunology in the world.

《肘后备急方》还提出"疠气"的病因,明确指出"家人视病者,亦可先服取利,则不相染易也"。这说明古人已经认识到疫病具有传染性,可以通过服用中药来预防疫病。

Also in Ge Hong's *Handbook of Prescriptions for Emergencies*, besides the source of the "epidemic pathogenic qi", it's stated that "If the family of the patient came to see him, the risk of infection could be minimized after having decoction of herbal medicine." These records indicated that in the early days, the ancients had gained the rising awareness of infectivity of the epidemic disease, and also the preventative measures by taking Chinese herbal decotion.

疟疾是对人类危害最大的疾病之一。青蒿素治疗疟疾的记载始于葛洪的《肘后备急方》。这部典籍首先提出了空气消毒法,用雄黄、雌黄、朱砂等为主的空气消毒药物制成太乙流金方、虎头杀鬼方等预防传染病的方剂。此外,《肘后备急方》还率先提出了井水消毒法。

Malaria is one of the most damaging diseases to mankind. The use of artemisinin to treat malaria begins with Ge's *Handbook of Prescriptions for Emergencies*, which also proposes air disinfection for the first time. This results in the creation of formulas such as *Taiyi Liujin* Formula and *Hutou Shagui* Formula in respect of prevention of infectious diseases mainly by using a combination of coexisting air disinfection medicine such as realgar, orpiment and cinnabar, etc. There is also the first mention of disinfection of well water in this classic.

南北朝时期,陈延之率先提出了"伤寒与天行瘟疫为异气"的观点,在其著作《小品方》中阐述了伤寒与时行瘟疫的区别。

During the Southern and Northern Dynasties, Chen Yanzhi was among the first to suggest the idea that "cold-induced febrile disease and pestilence are all pestilent *qi*". In his *Classical Prescriptions*, he went on to elaborate the distinction between cold-induced febrile disease and epidemic-prone pestilence.

第四章　唐宋时期

　　唐朝时期发生疫情，朝廷和地方官府都会采取一定的抗疫举措。唐文宗大和六年（公元832年），南方发生疾疫，朝廷专门颁布"拯恤疾疫诏"："自诸道水旱害人，疫疾相继，宵旰罪己，兴寝疚怀，屡降诏书，俾副勤恤。"朝廷还制定了疫病发生后的应对举措，"其疫未定处，并委长吏差官巡抚，量给医药，询问救疗之术，各加拯济"。

Chapter 4　Period of the Tang and Song Dynasties

　　During the Tang Dynasty, whenever there was epidemic outbreak, both the imperial court and local government would have certain anti-epidemic measures well planned. In the sixth Dahe year (832 A.D.) during the reign of the Tang Dynasty, Emperor Wenzong, a pestilence swept the southern part of the land. A special-purpose imperial edict, called "Edict for Relief of Victims of a Pestilence", was issued by the imperial court. "Ever since rampant floods and deadly droughts have troubled south, and pestilence has come in succession, I am guilt-ridden and couldn't sleep. I have issued edicts for the relief of the victims several times." The imperial court also tailored relief measures to tackle the worsening epidemic situation, "In areas with still unsettled epidemiological situation, officials were required to go on tours of inspection, mandating efforts to reduce the sufferings, enquiring cures for the patients, providing targeted medicine, and offering relief and support."

　　唐宋时期和疫病相关的代表性医著有王焘的《外台秘要》、孙思邈的《备急千金要方》、王怀隐等的《太平圣惠方》以及宋代太平惠民和剂局编写的《太平惠民和剂局方》等。

During the Tang and Song Dynasties, epidemic-related representative monumental medical works embraced *Arcane Essentials from the Imperial Library* by Wang Tao, *Prescriptions Worth a Thousand Pieces of Gold for Emergencies* by Sun Simiao, *Taiping Holy Prescriptions for Universal Relief* by Wang Huaiyin and *Formularies of the Bureau of Taiping People's Welfare Pharmacy*, etc.

《外台秘要》是唐朝一部综合性医学巨著,书中有对伤寒、肺结核、疟疾、天花、霍乱等传染病的描述,收载防治疫病的方剂数十首。《外台秘要》被历代医家誉为"世宝",世人普遍认为"不观《外台》方,不读《千金》论,则医人所见不广,用药不神"。

Arcane Essentials from the Imperial Library, a comprehensive monumental work of medicine in the Tang Dynasty, gave a general description of infectious diseases such as cold-induced febrile disease, tuberculosis, malaria, smallpox, cholera and so on, and embraced dozens of TCM formulae in epidemic disease control and prevention. This classic was acclaimed as a "World Treasure" by physicians through the ages. It was generally admitted that "Physicians will be short of deep insight and marvelous curative effect without reading *Arcane Essentials from the Imperial Library* and *Prescriptions Worth a Thousand Gold*."

唐代孙思邈所撰《备急千金要方》共载有 42 首辟瘟、治瘟成方,此书还提出用熏药法进行空气消毒,向井中投入药物给水消毒,将雄黄、朱砂作为消毒药物等消毒法。《备急千金要方》中还有佩"绎囊"和"避疫气,令人不染"的记载,指出佩戴香囊具有辟秽和预防传染的功效。《备急千金要方》还指出疫病"病从口入"的传播途径,"夫霍乱之病,皆因饮食,非关鬼神"。此外,《备急千金要方》还记载了饮用屠苏酒防疫的方法。

During the Tang Dynasty, formulae on prevention and treatment of epidemic diseases recorded in *Prescriptions Worth a Thousand Pieces of Gold for Emergencies* by Sun Simiao amounted to 42. Also this classic proposed multiple methods of disinfection, such as the use of Chinese herbal fumigation to sterilize the air, dropping medicine into wells to disinfect the water, and using realgar and cinnabar as disinfection medicine, etc. In *Prescriptions Worth a Thousand Gold for Emergencies*, it not only presented a record of wearing "scented sachet", but stated that "repelling evil pathogenic *qi* assists in reducing infection risks", making it clear that wearing scented sachet targeted to ward off filth and infection prevention. The transmission route of epidemic diseases, "disease entering by the mouth", was also made clear by this work, "Instead of ghosts and gods, diet is the biggest cause of cholera." *Tusu* wine, in addition, was recorded in this book as an assistant of epidemic prevention.

《太平圣惠方》是宋朝政府诏令集体编修的一部综合性医学巨著，历时14年，由翰林医官王怀隐等人负责。《太平圣惠方》涉及伤寒、时气、热病、霍乱等，载有许多治疗疫病的经验，内容极其丰富，故北宋著名书法家蔡襄曾赞《太平圣惠方》多异域瑰奇之品。

The comprehensive medical masterpiece, *Taiping Holy Prescriptions for Universal Relief* compiled collectively by Wang Huaiyin, the head of the Imperial Academy of Medicine, and other officials of the department under the command of the government in the Song Dynasty with 14 years' effort, was rich in content, bulging with descriptions of cold-induced febrile disease, pestilent epidemic *qi*, heat disease, cholera, and experiences on treatment of epidemic diseases. Cai Xiang, a renowned calligrapher in the Northern Song Dynasty, spoke in glowing terms of its content, brilliant and rare were used to describe this book.

宋朝时期，太平惠民和剂局编写的《太平惠民和剂局方》是我国医学史上第一部由国家颁行的成药标准和配方手册,在中医方剂学发展史上有举足轻重的地位。

During the Song Dynasty, *Formularies of the Bureau of Taiping People's Welfare Pharmacy*, compiled by Bureau for Taiping People's Welfare Pharmacy, was the first standard of patent medicine and formula manual issued by the government in the history of TCM. This book had a substantial carry-over impact on the history of the development of formulaology in TCM.

第五章　金朝时期

金朝时期，刘完素提出了以火热为主的病机观和以寒凉为主的治疗观。刘完素认为医学的精微要旨尽在《黄帝内经》之中，在《黄帝内经》"病机十九条"理论的基础之上，他提出了火热病症"火热为病"的观点。此外，他认为治疗温病用药应以寒凉为主。他的三部代表作为《素问玄机原病式》《黄帝素问宣明论方》和《素问病机气宜保命集》。

Chapter 5　Period of the Jin Dynasty

During the Jin Dynasty, Liu Wansu presented his two-fold viewpoint: fire-heat syndrome in pathogenesis and cold-cool medication in treatment. Liu Wansu deemed that *Inner Canon of the Yellow Emperor* wrapped up all its essentials and subtleties of medicine. Based on the theory of "19 items of pathogenesis" in this classic, he made point of "fire and heat causing disease" in fire-heat syndrome treatment. What's more, he considered drugs cold and cool were mostly employed for clinical treatment of warm disease. Three most representative works of Liu Wansu were *Exploration to Mysterious Pathogenesis and Etiology Based on Plain Questions*, *Prescriptions and Exposition of Huangdi's Plain Questions* and *Collection of Writings on the Mechanism of Disease*, *Suitability of Qi and Safeguarding of Life Discussed in Plain Questions*.

张从正认为病由邪生，治病当先攻邪，邪气除尽则正气自复。发汗、催吐、泻下是攻邪的三大治法。

Zhang Congzheng raised the idea of diseases arising from pathogens and attacking pathogens first in treating disease. The vital healthy *qi* would be exuberant only after the pathogenic evil *qi* was firstly eliminated. Inducing sweat, promoting emesis, and purgation were three major methods employed by Zhang Congzheng to eliminate pathogens.

作为脾胃学说的创始人,李杲的代表作有《内外伤辨惑论》《脾胃论》《兰室秘藏》等。李杲生活的年代战乱、瘟疫不断,他创制"普济消毒饮"用于治疗一种名叫"大头瘟"的急性传染病,疗效显著。

As the founder of spleen and stomach theory, Li Gao wrote much, among which were *Treatise on Classification of Perplexities about Internal and External Damage*, *Treatise on Spleen and Stomach* and *Secret Book of the Orchid Chamber*. The age in which he lived was hit hard by war and pestilence, which spurred his creation of Universal Relief Disinfection Decoction to treat an acute infectious disease known as "Swollen-Head Infection" with remarkable effectiveness.

第六章　元明清时期

元朝朱震亨创立"滋阴派",奠定了滋阴降火学说的理论基础,促进了明清温热学说的形成和发展。

Chapter 6　Period of the Yuan, Ming and Qing Dynasties

During the Yuan Dynasty, Zhu Zhenheng created school of "nourishing yin", which established the theoretical basis for theory of "nourishing yin to reduce fire" and facilitated the formation and development of the theory of "warm heat" during the Ming and Qing Dynasties.

明朝李时珍所撰《本草纲目》记载了蒸煮消毒、空气消毒、食醋消毒等多种防疫方法。在空气消毒方面,可于房内焚烧苍术、艾叶、白芷、丁香、硫黄等药进行空气消毒辟秽。在高温蒸煮消毒方面,《本草纲目》记载:"天行疫瘟,取初病患衣服,于甑上蒸过,则一家不染。"

In the Ming Dynasty, Li Shizhen, a legendary Chinese pharmacist in the 16th century, set aside methods of epidemic prevention such as steaming and boiling disinfection, air disinfection and vinegar disinfection in his work *Compendium of Materia Medica*. In terms of air disinfection, according to this classic, atractylodes rhizome, artemisia argyi, angelica dahurica, clove and sulphur could be burned to repel the evil pathogenic *qi*. Records from *Compendium of Materia Medica* stated that "In respect of steaming and boiling disinfection, there wouldn't a sign of infection when the patient's clothes and bedding got steamed and boiled on an ancient earthen utensil for steaming at the instant of pestilence occurrence."

明朝时期,出现了预防天花的人痘接种术,这是世界上最早的疫苗雏形,成为人工免疫的先驱。人痘接种术源于中国,后经阿拉伯、土耳其传入欧洲。明清时期已有以种痘为业的专职痘医,清代政府还专门设有种痘局,向民众普及种痘,这是世界上最早的免疫机构。清代宫廷曾设避痘所来隔离感染天花者。

Variolation appeared in the Ming Dynasty, which served as the world's earliest embryonic vaccine against smallpox and undoubtedly pioneered artificial immunity. Variolation, originated in China and developed in Arab countries and Turkey later on, was finally introduced to Europe through these countries. In the Ming and Qing Dynasties, professional doctors for vaccination arose. During the Qing Dynasty, Bureau for Vaccination, the world's earliest immunization organization, was set up to popularize vaccination, and Vaccination Prevention Site against smallpox was established in the royal court to make the infected people in quarantine.

明清时期,温病学说的形成与发展是中医学理论的一大突破。1642 年,吴又可编著《温疫论》,对温病学说的创立起到了促进作用。《温疫论》是中国历史上第一部系统研究急性传染病的医学著作。《温疫论》提出传染病的病因观——"戾气"学说,指出传染病的主要传染途径为自"口鼻而入"。吴又可认为瘟疫有极强的传染性,"无问老幼,触者皆病"。在我国明朝没有显微镜的时代背景下,吴又可科学预见了细菌、病毒等致病微生物的存在,并且提出了实用方剂——达原饮。

During the Ming and Qing Dynasties, the formation and development of the warm disease theory was a breakthrough in the theory of Chinese medicine. *Treatise on Pestilence*, compiled in 1642 by Wu Youke, played a stimulative role in the creation of warm disease theory. *Treatise on Pestilence* was the first medical book specializing in acute infectious disease in China. Not only did it advance the etiology of infectious disease—the theory of "epidemic pestilential qi", it also pointed out the main transmission routes of infection—mouth and nose. Wu Youke deemed that pestilence was highly contagious, "Once contacted, all ages, old and young, were stricken with the infectious disease." Under the background of the absence of microscopes in the Ming Dynasty in China, Wu

Youke foresaw the existence of pathogenic microorganism such as bacteria and viruses scientifically. The practical formula—*Dayuan* Decoction was also unveiled by him.

至清代，中医在疫病的治疗方面积累了丰富的经验，相关著述可谓汗牛充栋。1746 年，叶天士著《温热论》，创温病的卫气营血辨证理论，系统分析了温热病的病理、诊断方法和治法，指出"温邪上受，首先犯肺"，温病学说创立。1799 年，吴鞠通著《温病条辨》，创温病学三焦辨证理论，确立了清热养阴的治疗原则。这些专著总结了防治温病的经验，在理论上颇有建树。除此之外，其他代表作还有薛生白的《湿热条辨》、王士雄的《温热经纬》和《霍乱论》、余霖的《疫疹一得》、戴天章的《广瘟疫论》、杨栗山的《伤寒温疫条辨》、刘松峰的《松峰说疫》、李炳的《辨疫琐言》、吴宣崇的《治鼠疫法》（中国第一部防治鼠疫的专著）、郑肖岩的《鼠疫约编》、罗汝兰的《鼠疫汇编》、喻嘉言的《寓意草》（载有人工种痘法）等。

By the Qing Dynasty, TCM had accumulated rich experiences in treating epidemic diseases and relevant clustered writings were immense. In 1746, *Treatise on Warm Febrile Diseases* by Ye Tianshi, which gave systematic analysis of the pathology, ways of diagnosis and treatment of warm febrile diseases, created therapies for such diseases based on syndrome differentiation system by adopting the defensive, *qi*, nutritive and blood as a theoretical model, thus urging the creation of the theory of warm disease. This classic further pinpointed that "As the spread of the pathogenic warmth, the lung becomes the prime target for attack." In 1799, *Treatise on Differentiation and Treatment of Warm Diseases* by Wu Jutong created triple-energizer syndrome differentiation and treatment on warm diseases, and established therapeutic principle of clearing heat and nourishing yin. These monographs yielded fruitful results in theory in this field with summing up experiences on warm diseases prevention and control. In addition, other representative works embraced *Treatise on Differentiation and Treatment of Pathogenic Dampness-Heat Diseases* by Xue Shengbai, *An Outline of Warm-Heat Diseases* and *Discussion on Cholera* by Wang Shixiong, *Yizhen Yide* by Yu Lin, *Treatise on Widespread Pestilence* by Dai Tianzhang, *Treatise on Differentiation and*

Treatment of Febrile Disease and Pestilence by Yang Lishan, *On Epidemics by Songfeng* by Liu Songfeng and *Trifle Talks in Differentiation of Epidemic* by Li Bing, *Method for Prevention and Treatment of Plague* (the first plague prevention and control monograph in China) by Wu Xuanchong, *Collection of Plague* by Zheng Xiaoyan, *A Corpus of Plague* by Luo Rulan, *Symbolized Grass* by Yu Jiayan with a record of variolation, etc.

据王士雄的《霍乱论》记载："人烟稠密之区,疫疠流行。"王士雄认为,人员密集的地方,疫病传播的可能性会加大,这与现在倡导的疫病流行期间不宜聚众集会的观点是一致的。

In Wang Shixiong's *Discussion on Cholera*, he wrote that "Densely populated areas tend to trigger epidemic disease." He expressed the opinion that crowded places increased the possibility of epidemic disease transmission, which was in line with today's advocating of less gathering during outbreaks of epidemic diseases.

1910年,东北发生鼠疫,中国检疫、防疫事业的先驱伍连德主持防疫工作。伍连德认为这场鼠疫可通过呼吸传染,人际传播是主要渠道,因此采取了大规模的隔离防疫措施,并且强制要求人们佩戴口罩。1911年,我国历史上第一次国际医学会议——"万国鼠疫研究会"召开,"北满防疫处"由此成立。

In the late Qing Dynasty, a plague swept across northeast China in 1910. Wu Lien-Teh, a pioneer for the cause of quarantine and anti-epidemic in China, presided over the anti-epidemic campaign. That plague, which he deemed as a highly contagious respiratory disease, spread mainly by person-to-person transmission. Hence large-scale response quarantine measures were implemented, and the government decided to make it mandatory for potential reservoirs of infection to wear masks. In 1911, "International Plague Conference" was held and became the first-ever gathering international medical science academic conference with the theme of plague prevention and control in China, which yielded the most important outcome of this conference—"Beiman Plague Prevention Bureau".

第七章　近现代时期

1950年，第一届全国卫生工作会议在北京召开，此次会议确立了"预防为主""团结中西医"的卫生工作方针。

Chapter 7　Period of Modern and Contemporary Times

In 1950, the first session of Public Health Work Conference was held in Beijing, which established "Prevention First" and "Combining Chinese and Western Medicine" as the guidelines for health work.

1956年，石家庄暴发流行性乙型脑炎，中药汤剂白虎汤大见奇效，治愈了90%以上的患者。

An epidemic encephalitis B swept north China's Shijiazhuang City in 1956. Chinese materia medica decoction, *Baihu* Decoction grappled with the encephalitis and made miraculous effect. The cure rate for the encephalitis patients was over 90 percent.

1967年5月23日，中国政府在北京启动"523"项目，研发新的抗疟药物。屠呦呦从《肘后备急方》中获取灵感，带领团队筛选出青蒿作为抗疟首选药物。

The Chinese government launched "523" project, a concerted national effort to discover a new treatment for malaria on May 23, 1967 in Beijing. Inspired by *Handbook of Prescriptions for Emergencies*, Tu Youyou filtered out *qinghao* (sweet wormwood shrub) as the top priority for anti-malaria treatment with her team.

2003 年,中医药抗击非典型性肺炎再立新功,国医大师邓铁涛推动中医药抗击非典,创造了零死亡、零感染、零后遗症的奇迹。中医药的治疗效果得到了世界卫生组织的肯定和赞扬。2004 年,我国出台了《传染性非典型肺炎(SARS)诊疗方案(2004 版)》。

In 2003, TCM rose to new contributions for its role in curbing the spread of Severe Acute Respiratory Syndrome (SARS). Deng Tietao, a famous TCM master, pushed TCM forward to perform miracles of zero death, zero new infections and zero sequelae. The therapeutic effect of TCM was affirmed and praised by the World Health Organization. "Diagnosis and Treatment Protocol for Severe Acute Respiratory Syndrome (Version 2004)" was released in 2004.

2009 年,甲型 H1N1 流感来袭,中医药优选出抗击疫情的方剂——金花清感方。金花清感颗粒是甲型 H1N1 流感流行期间研发的中成药,由金银花、薄荷、甘草等 12 味药组成,疗效确切。

During the H1N1 influenza outbreak in 2009, TCM joint the fight again and *Jinhua Qinggan* Prescription was optimized. *Jinhua Qinggan* Granule, which contained 12 herbal components involving honeysuckle, mint, licorice and so on, was developed during the pandemic as it previously proved to be effective in the battle against the H1N1 influenza.

自新冠肺炎疫情暴发以来,中国采取了坚决的措施防控疫情。通过临床筛选出的"三药三方"书写了中药抗疫方案,疗效确切。"三药"即金花清感颗粒、连花清瘟胶囊、血必净注射液。"三方"是指清肺排毒汤、化湿败毒方、宣肺败毒方三个方剂。其中,清肺排毒汤源自张仲景所著《伤寒杂病论》,由几个经典方剂融合而成,全方共含 21 味中药成分。《新型冠状病毒肺炎诊疗方案(试行第七版)》将清肺排毒汤列为中医临床治疗药物的首选。2020 年 2 月 12 日,张伯礼率领中医医疗团队进驻江夏方舱医院,这是中华人民共和国成立以来中医第一次独立运营的一家传染病医院。在抗击新冠肺炎疫情中,中医药再次发挥了重要作用。

Since the outbreak of coronavirus disease (COVID-19), China has launched a resolute battle to prevent and control its spread. TCM again is on the front line, fighting with virus. Three TCM prescriptions and three anti-epidemic drugs have been proved by clinical data to show curative effects in treatment, including *Jinhua Qinggan* Granule, *Lianhua Qingwen* Capsule, *Xuebijing* Injection, Lung Cleansing and Detoxifying Decoction, Huashi Baidu Formula and *Xuanfei Baidu* Formula. Lung Cleansing and Detoxifying Decoction, which has 21 herbal ingredients, comes from fusions of several classic formulae in *Treatise on Febrile Diseases and Miscellaneous Illnesses* by Zhang Zhongjing. According to "Diagnosis and Treatment Protocol for COVID-19 (Trial Version 7)" published by National Health Commission of the People's Republic of China, Lung Cleansing and Detoxifying Decoction ranks first among TCM clinical therapeutic solutions. On February 12, 2020, a TCM medical team led by Zhang Boli, moved into Jiangxia Fangcang Makeshift Hospital, which served as China's first independent operated makeshift hospital featuring traditional Chinese medicine to treat COVID-19 patients. TCM rose to public prominence for its big role in China's fight against the coronavirus.

纵观历史,抗击新冠肺炎疫情的实践再次充分证明,中医药以前是,现在是,未来仍然是人类与疫病斗争的重要武器。

A review of the history and China's fight against coronavirus disease (COVID-19) fully reveals a fact again: TCM, the time-tested cure, is still mankind's powerful weapon against epidemic diseases in the past, present, and future.

参考文献
Bibliography

[1] 班固. 汉书[M]. 北京:中华书局,2007.
[2] 曹雪芹. 红楼梦[M]. 俞平伯,校;启功,注. 北京:人民文学出版社,2020.
[3] 陈元龙. 格致镜原[M]. 扬州:广陵古籍刻印社,1989.
[4] 大中华文库汉英对照:吕氏春秋[M]. 翟江月,译. 桂林:广西师范大学出版社,2005.
[5] 大中华文库汉英对照:尚书[M]. 周秉钧,今译;理雅各,英译. 长沙:湖南人民出版社,2013.
[6] 大中华文库汉英对照:荀子[M]. 张觉,今译;约翰·诺布洛克,英译. 长沙:湖南人民出版社,1999.
[7] 大中华文库汉英对照:周易[M]. 傅惠生,英译;张善文,今译. 长沙:湖南人民出版社,2008.
[8] 戴圣. 礼记[M]. 陈澔,注;金晓东,点校. 上海:上海古籍出版社,2016.
[9] 葛洪. 肘后备急方[M]. 王均宁,点校. 天津:天津科学技术出版社,2005.
[10] 龚廷贤. 龚廷贤医学全书[M]. 太原:山西科学技术出版社,2016.
[11] 韩非. 韩非子[M]. 王先慎,集解;姜俊俊,点校. 上海:上海古籍出版社,2015.
[12] 淮南子[M]. 顾迁,译注. 北京:中华书局,2009.
[13] 黄帝内经[M]. 姚春鹏,注. 北京:中华书局,2009.
[14] 黄帝内经·灵枢[M]. 刘希茹,李照国,译注. 西安:世界图书出版西安公司,2008.
[15] 黄帝内经·素问[M]. 刘希茹,李照国,译注. 西安:世界图书出版西安公司,2005.
[16] 林语堂. 老子的智慧[M]. 合肥:安徽科学技术出版社,2012.

[17] 凌耀星. 中医古籍整理丛书重刊·难经校注[M]. 北京:人民卫生出版社,2013.
[18] 刘宁,刘景源. 中医千年抗疫史及新冠肺炎研究与思考[M]. 北京:中国中医药出版社,2020.
[19] 山海经[M]. 方韬,译注. 北京:中华书局,2011.
[20] 许浩. 复斋日记[M]. 北京:商务印书馆,1936.
[21] 许慎. 说文解字注[M]. 段玉裁,注. 上海:上海古籍出版社,1981.
[22] 荀况. 荀子[M]. 安小兰,译注. 北京:中华书局,2007.
[23] 杨伯峻. 春秋左传注[M]. 北京:中华书局,2016.
[24] 喻昌. 医门法律[M]. 史欣德,整理. 北京:人民卫生出版社,2006.
[25] 张介宾. 类经[M]. 郭洪耀,吴少祯,校注. 北京:中国中医药出版社,1997.
[26] 中国中医研究院. 中国疫病史鉴[M]. 北京:中医古籍出版社,2003.
[27] 周公旦. 周礼[M]. 徐正英,常佩雨,译注. 北京:中华书局,2014.
[28] 朱震亨. 丹溪心法[M]. 王英,竹剑平,江凌圳,整理. 北京:人民卫生出版社,2005.
[29] 左丘明. 左传[M]. 郭丹,程小青,李彬源,译注. 北京:中华书局,2016.

附录1：常见中医典籍名称中英文对照表
Appendix 1: Common Chinese-English Titles of TCM Classics

B

《备急千金要方》*Prescriptions Worth a Thousand Pieces of Gold for Emergencies*
《本草纲目》*Compendium of Materia Medica*

H

《黄帝内经》*Inner Canon of the Yellow Emperor*
《黄帝内经·灵枢》*Spiritual Pivot*
《黄帝内经·素问》*Plain Questions*

L

《类经》*The Classified Classic*

N

《难经》*Classic of Medical Difficulties*

S

《伤寒杂病论》*Treatise on Febrile Diseases and Miscellaneous Illnesses*
《神农本草经》*Shennong's Classic of Materia Medica*

W

《温热论》*Treatise on Warm Febrile Diseases*

Z

《针灸甲乙经》*A-B Canon of Acupuncture and Moxibustion*
《肘后备急方》*Handbook of Prescriptions for Emergencies*
《诸病源候论》*Treatise on Causes and Symptoms of Diseases*

附录2：中医常用术语中英文对照表
Appendix 2: Commonly Used Terminologies of TCM

B

辨证论治 treatment based on syndrome differentiation

D

大肠 large intestine
大怒伤肝 great anger impairing the liver
胆 gallbladder
胆气 gallbladder *qi*
胆汁 bile
胆主决断 The gallbladder is associated with decision making and judgment.

F

方剂 prescription

肺气 lung *qi*

肺阳 lung yang

肺阴 lung yin

肺主皮毛 The lung governs the skin and hair.

肺主气 The lung governs *qi*.

肺主肃降 The lung governs depuration and descent.

肺主通调水道 The lung governs regulation of water passage.

肺主宣发 The lung governs dispersion.

肺主治节 The lung governs management and regulation.

风寒感冒 common cold due to wind and cold

G

肝气 liver *qi*

肝气上逆 ascending counter-flow of liver *qi*

肝肾同源 The liver and the kidney are of the same origin.

肝血 liver blood

肝阳 liver yang

肝阴 liver yin

肝主藏血 The liver stores the blood.

肝主疏泄 The liver governs coursing and discharge.

孤腑 solitary *fu*-organ

J

金水相生 generation between metal and water

津血同源 Body fluid and blood share the same origin.

经络系统 system of meridians and collaterals

经络学说 theory of meridians and collaterals

精气 essential *qi*

K

开胃消食 stimulate appetite and promote digestion

L

临床经验 clinical experience

临床实践 clinical practice
六腑 six *fu*-organs

M

脉象细弱 thin and weak pulse
面色红润 rosy complexion
面色无华 lusterless complexion
命门 life gate
母病及子 disorder of a mother-organ involving its child-organ

P

脾气 spleen *qi*
脾胃虚弱 weakness of the spleen and stomach
脾阳 spleen yang
脾阴 spleen yin
脾主升清 The spleen governs ascent of the clear.
脾主统血 The spleen controls the blood.
脾主运化 The spleen governs transportation and transformation.

Q

奇恒之腑 extraordinary *fu*-organs

气化 *qi* transformation

气机 *qi* movement

七情内伤 internal injury by seven emotions

气为血帅 *qi* as the commander of the blood

气虚 *qi* deficiency

气滞血瘀 stagnation of *qi* and blood stasis

S

三焦 triple energizer

肾藏精 The kidney stores essence.

肾精 kidney essence

肾气 kidney *qi*

肾阳 kidney yang

肾阴 kidney yin

肾阴不足 insufficiency of kidney yin

肾主纳气 The kidney governs reception of *qi*.

肾主水 The kidney governs water.

升降出入 ascending, descending, exiting and entering

生克制化 generation and restriction

四气五味 four properties and five tastes

四诊法 four diagnostic methods

四诊合参 comprehensive analysis by the four diagnostic methods

T

天人合一 Man and nature are united as one.

天人相应 correspondence between man and the nature

同病异治 treat the same disease with different therapies

W

望闻问切 inspection, auscultation and olfaction, inquiry, pulse-taking and palpation

卫气 defense *qi*

胃气 stomach *qi*

胃阳 stomach yang

胃阴 stomach yin

胃主腐熟 The stomach governs decomposition.

胃主受纳 The stomach governs intake.

胃主通降 The stomach governs descent.

五行 five elements

五行相乘 over-restriction among the five elements

五行相克 restriction among the five elements

五行相生 generation among the five elements

五行相侮 counter-restriction among the five elements

五行学说 theory of the five elements

五运 five circuits

五脏 five *zang*-organs

五行制化 inhibition and transformation among the five elements

X

相克 restriction

相生 generation

小肠 small intestine

心气 heart *qi*

心气充沛 sufficiency of heart *qi*

心血 heart blood

心阳 heart yang

心阴 heart yin

心主神明 The heart governs the mind.

心主血脉 The heart governs the blood and vessels.

Y

阳气 yang *qi*

异病同治 treat different diseases with the same therapy

阴平阳秘 Yin is stable and yang is compact.

阴气 yin *qi*

阴阳 yin and yang

阴阳互根 mutual rooting of yin and yang

阴阳交感 interaction of yin and yang

阴阳消长 waxing and waning of yin and yang

阴阳转化 mutual conversion of yin and yang

阴阳自和 spontaneous harmonization of yin and yang

营气 nutrient *qi*

元气 original *qi*

元气充盈 sufficiency of the original *qi*

元气耗伤 decline of the original *qi*

Z

杂病 miscellaneous diseases

脏腑 *zang-fu* organs

藏象 visceral manifestation

藏象学说 theory of visceral manifestation

针灸 acupuncture and moxibustion

整体观念 holism

主气 dominant *qi*

滋阴降火 nourishing yin and reducing fire

后 记
Afterword

  本书在编写过程中得到了河南中医药大学校办、团委及各部门的鼎力协助。人物肖像为校书画院副院长王振超所绘,古籍图片由图书馆古籍部提供,中药传奇篇的图片由药学院董诚明副院长和杨晶凡老师提供,其他图片由医史馆、仲景馆和抗疫馆提供,谨致谢忱。